MY GRAIN
&BRAIN
GLUTEN-FREE
SLOW COOKER
COOKBOOK

MY GRAIN & BRAIN GLUTEN-FREE SLOW COOKER COOKBOOK

Brain Healthy and Grain-free Slow Cooker Recipes Everyone Can Use To Boost Brain Power, Lose Belly Fat and Live Healthy - A Gluten-free, Low Sugar, Low Carb and Wheat-Free Slow Cooker Cookbook

SHERYL JENSEN

DISCLAIMER

The information provided in this book is for educational purposes only. I am not a physician and this is not to be taken as medical advice or a recommendation to stop eating other foods. This book is based on my experiences and interpretations of the past and current research available. If you have any health issues or pre-existing conditions, please consult your doctor before implementing any of the information that is presented in this book. Results may vary from individual to individual. This book is for informational purposes only and the author does not accept any responsibilities for any liabilities or damages, real or perceived, resulting from the use of this information.

TABLE OF CONTENTS

A GLUTEN-FREE JOURNEY WORTH TAKING

"Enjoy gluten-free slow cooked meals while you improve your brain health, lose weight and optimize your overall health – that's what you'll get from the gluten-free recipes in My Grain & Brain Gluten-free Slow Cooker Cookbook"

You are not alone if you get up some mornings and just wished that your breakfast was waiting for you. Or maybe after a busy day at work, you get home in the evening and just wished that dinner was ready. Well, your solution is right here for your taking. Now you can prepare your meals ahead of time and enjoy a healthy gluten-free meal just when you need it. It is indeed a beautiful experience to have a warm, healthy and delicious meal waiting for you in your slow cooker.

Moreover, cooking gluten-free does not only become easier and healthier with your slow cooker, but it also becomes more affordable. With your slow cooker you'll be able to convert a budget-cut meat into a healthy and succulent meal. Therefore, if you've started the gluten-free journey and you think that you don't have the time to stick to it, making use of a slow-cooker is your next best option.

This specially created cookbook collection boasts over 100 of the healthiest and easiest gluten-free slow cooker recipes. Your grain and brain journey would not be complete without trying your hand with these gluten-free slow cooker recipes. Whether you are a busy person or not, you wouldn't want to miss these slow cooker recipes. Now you can start or maintain your brain healthy gluten-free diet without worrying about time constraints. Following a brain healthy diet just got easier!

THE GRAIN BLAME REALITY

Let's back track a bit. The truth is that we've been taught the wrong stuff about gluten over the decades. It all started centuries ago with the Egyptians. The Egyptians were the ones who started to store grains and use it as a contingency plan for times of drought and famine. In the interim, the use of non-genetically modified wheat in those challenging times had saved a lot of lives. Centuries later manufacturers of genetically modified wheat and grains jumped on the bandwagon and as a result, we've been experiencing the overwhelming distress of gluten ever since.

What Makes Gluten A Problem?

Gluten consumption has justifiably become increasingly popular over the last decades. And no wonder – gluten, the unhealthy protein component that is found in processed wheat and other grains is available in an alarming variety of processed foods and even medications.

Simply put, there is a protein that is in grains such as wheat, oat, barley and rye. This protein is commonly mentioned as gluten. Now, this complex gluten protein is very difficult for our stomachs to digest. Usually, these difficult to digest complex protein will remain undigested in the body and triggers a host of other problems in the process. Of course, these digestive problems will have a negative impact on our health and often triggers tissue destruction related intestinal problems such as Celiac Disease, Collitis, Irritable Bowel Syndrome, Chron's Disease and other chronic diseases. Furthermore, gluten sensitivity adversely affects our tissues and nervous system and is not always an intestinal problem. Consequently, cases of gluten sensitivity often go on to produce neurological symptoms.

The health benefits of living without gluten are increasingly becoming widely acknowledged by scientists and doctors alike. Based on much scientific and medical evidence, life without gluten has many potential benefits, such as:

- Improved brain health

- Weight loss
- Improvement in gastrointestinal problems
- Increased energy
- Reduced bloating and gas
- Decreased risk of heart disease
- Improvement in allergy control
- Decreased cancer risk
- Improvement in symptoms of Celiac disease
- Reduced risk or improvement of diabetes
- Plus improvement in overall health

Grain and Brain

For some time, the terms *"grain" and "brain"* have been widely used to refer to the correlation between grain consumption and brain health. Today, statistical data have confirmed that there has been a significant increase of neurological disorders as mild as brain fog or as severe as Alzheimer's disease, childhood development disorders, Parkinson's, autism, dementia, multiple sclerosis and other brain related neurogenerative disorders. As a result, various laboratory studies have been conducted to assist in identifying the cause of such a significant surge.

Increasingly, different laboratory findings have already confirmed that by eliminating gluten from the diet there has been an overwhelmingly positive effect on the brain health of many people. In fact, even a recent analysis study that was conducted by well-known immunologist, Aristo Vojdani (PhD). Based on blood samples from 400 healthy people, it was revealed that there is a substantial connection between gluten consumption and neurological autoimmunity or reaction.

Based on the adverse reactions of gluten in the body, there is some form of "tagging" going on in the immune system in order to destroy complex gluten molecules. However, according to studies by immunologist, Aristo Vojdani, PhD and others, as in a case of mistaken identity, the immune system mistakably attacks and also destroys brain and nerve tissue while discerning that it is attacking the gluten. So in other words, gluten consumption is causing your immune system to mistakenly attack and destroy your brain. Interesting? Isn't it!

Consider that if you've done tests that reveal that you're gluten sensitive you should adapt a gluten-free diet as quickly as possible. However, also bear in mind, that based on current gluten sensitivity tests, your sensitivity to gluten could go undetected for several years, even though gluten could still be negatively affecting your health.

So whether you've been diagnosed with gluten sensitivities or not, you should avoid gluten at all cost. Besides, many people who have adapted a gluten-free lifestyle have reported significant weight loss results and an overall improvement in their health. Save your brain and your health—go gluten-free!

GLUTEN-FREE FOR BEGINNERS

If you're already familiar with living gluten-free you may skip this section and go right into the healthy gluten-free recipes. However, if you are new to the gluten-free lifestyle, you may find this section to be quite useful.

Gluten-free Shopping

You're advised to go shopping before you start your exciting gluten-free lifestyle. Preparation is essentially worth the effort and will make things so much easier. This will avoid you winding up in a frustrating situation where you are left with little or no options. Besides, lack of planning is the main reason for failures in life.

Before you go shopping, you can make a note of ingredients in the recipes that you will be preparing for a week or so. Your shopping list should be primarily based on the ingredients in the recipes. You should carefully create a shopping list before you head to the food store. Apart from the specific ingredients of the recipes, your list should always include ingredient extras and snacks. Please take a look at the 14 foods list guide in this book.

You will also need to clear your kitchen cabinets and refrigerator of the items that are not a part of the gluten-free diet or items that will not positively contribute to your gluten-free lifestyle. In doing so, you will need to get rid of bad fats, carbs and sugars so that you won't accidentally add them to a recipe or even feel tempted to use them.

Choosing your Food

Whenever you go gluten-free shopping you should ensure that you buy antibiotic-free and hormone-free animal, poultry, fish and red meat. You should look for free-range poultry and eggs as well as grass-fed beef, organic pork, wild fish or grass-fed butter. It is also important to choose freshly frozen meat which is also referred to as "flash" frozen.

You must also exercise caution when buying fruits, vegetables and nuts. Make an effort to buy fresh seasonal local vegetables and fruits that are certified to be organic. If you decide to get frozen fruits, you should ensure that they are free from added sugar. On the other hand, nuts should be raw and organic—most are welcome EXCEPT peanuts. Peanuts are not really "nuts" and can be potentially harmful due to their ability to pull essential minerals away from the body. Pecans, walnuts, and almonds are great for snacking.

Though organic food is generally more expensive, the benefits far outweigh the cost. Organic food contains lower levels of pesticides, hormones, and antibiotics than conventional foods. Furthermore, studies have also revealed that organic foods also have more nutrients when compared to foods grown conventionally.

Essential Gluten-free Kitchen Tools

There are several essential tools that could make your gluten-free lifestyle much easier. Though not all of these items are needed for the recipes in this book, they are simply essential items that you'll find useful in your gluten-free kitchen.

Apart from your slow cooker, here is a list of some other common essential gluten-free kitchen tools:

- A food processor
- A ladle
- A colander
- Ziplock storage bags of different sizes
- A powerful blender
- A dutch oven
- A grill pan
- A set of good-quality knives
- Wooden cutting boards—use separate boards for animal

- products and fruits or vegetables
- An 8-inch nonstick sauté pan
- A 12-inch nonstick sauté pan (avoid non-stick pans with Teflon or other health risks due to poorer quality)
- An 8-quart stockpot
- Cooling rack
- 3 or 4 cookie or baking sheets
- Oven mittens
- Storage glass jars for condiments
- Natural parchment paper
- A lemon/citrus reamer
- A food mill/potato ricer
- A 2-quart saucepan with lid
- A 4-quart saucepan with lid
- A foil lined baking tray
- A coffee grinder for flaxseed or similar stuff
- Wire whisks
- Spring tongs
- Rubber spatulas
- Assorted measuring cups and spoons (1 quart, pint, 1 cup etc.) dry and liquid style
- A food scale
- Muffin pans
- Baking pans
- Skewers
- An instant-read chef's thermometer
- Timer
- Mixing bowls of different sizes
- Electric mixer

Consider that this is not a conclusive list. Besides, you may already have some of these items in your kitchen.

SLOW COOKER FOR BEGINNERS

If you are already quite familiar with slow-cooking, then you may consider skipping this section and go straight into the recipes. For most people though, the slow cooker is mainly for cooking beans and soup dishes. But the fact is, you may cook many interesting dishes in the crock pot, ranging from breakfasts to even desserts—all gluten-free.

Knowing some simple little tips is essential for creating healthy and fulfilling slow-cooked meals. By following these few tips you'll be able to easily prepare tasty and healthy gluten-free slow cooker recipes anytime.

1. Sometimes browning your meat before putting it in the slow cooker is a good idea. Browning your meat usually helps to retain the flavor of the food.

2. Cutting your meats into bite-sized pieces will help to ensure that it will cook evenly and at the same time.

3. Slow cookers call for about 50% less liquid than the amount used in conventional cooking recipes.

4. Food won't cook properly in the slow cooker if there is too much or too little food. Therefore, ensure that your slow cooker is ½ to 2/3 full of food.

5. Your slow cooker responds differently to different cuts of meat. Usually, meats that are tough and thick become very tender on slow cooker's low heat while meats that are lean become very dry. Also, chicken cuts such as legs and thighs tend to retain more moisture than the whiter parts such as the breasts.

6. Even though stirring may be tempting, stirring is hardly necessary with the slow cooker.

7. Generally, 1 hour on high temperature would give the same result as 2 hours on low temperature.
8. Always cook with the cover on, but if you must peak, do so quickly. It may take up to 20 minutes to recover lost heat after you've removed the cover.
9. By nature, slow cookers cook food slower. For this reason, the flavors of seasonings may diminish. To counteract this issue ensure that you season your food liberally. You may add a little more fresh or dried herb during the last hour of cooking in order to maintain a stronger flavor.
10. Before serving food from your slow cooker always check the flavor of your food and adjust the taste with seasonings if necessary.
11. Never use frozen ingredients. Frozen food takes longer to cook and increases the possibility of harmful bacteria growth.
12. Unless you are following a specific recipe, be mindful that some ingredients such as milk, yogurt or cheese may spoil if they are not added at the right time. If in doubt, it is best to add these ingredients during the last hour of cooking.
13. For food safety purposes, a good slow cooker should reach a temperature of about 140 degrees Fahrenheit in at least 4 hours.
14. Slow cookers which are made of ceramic and glass material can crack or break. Do not add cold ingredients if the container or lid is hot. Neither should you put a hot container made of glass or ceramic material on a cold surface.
15. If you return home and realize that there was a power outage during your slow-cooking session, it is best that you discard the slow cooked food even if it seems fine. If you are at home during a power outage you may consider cooking the food by other means where possible.
16. In cases where you intend to re-heat leftovers from a slow-cooked meal, do not do your reheating in the slow cooker. Instead, you should transfer the leftovers to the microwave, stove or another suitable appliance.

Gluten-free Living Just Got Easier

Sadly, many people have misconceptions about going gluten-free, believing it is difficult to prepare and cook gluten-free. This is not entirely true, going gluten-free can be a stressful task, especially for beginners, but sometimes even for those who are already living the gluten-free lifestyle. However, it can become surprisingly simple if you follow the instructions given in the following pages. So, whether you are a total gluten-free newbie or not, your gluten-free journey can be so much easier with this gluten-free slow cooker cookbook.

This book consists of over 100 specially created, healthy and tasty gluten-free recipes. Apart from being gluten-free, these recipes are also wheat-free, low sugar, low carb and peanut-free. The choices of ingredients used in these recipes were carefully chosen, based on concrete scientific and medical research for a healthy gluten-free diet. Consequently, only the healthiest proteins, fats, fruits and vegetables are used in this book in order to ensure that you're eating to get the healthiest advantage.

Who Can Use These Recipes?

Broadly speaking, these recipes are for everyone who wants to use their slow cooker to prepare brain healthy foods, lose weight and live a healthy life. Even more specifically, these recipes are for you if you are looking for:

- Gluten-free Slow Cooker Recipes
- Gluten-free Recipes
- Grain-free Recipes
- Brain Healthy Recipes
- Wheat-free Recipes
- Immune System Boosting Recipes
- Celiac-friendly Recipes
- Autoimmune-friendly Recipes
- Diabetic-friendly Recipes
- Low Sugar Recipes
- Protein-rich Recipes
- Low Carb Recipes
- Soy-free Recipes
- Peanut-free Recipes

LET'S GET STARTED

In my slow cooker cookbook, you'll be able to prepare healthy and mouthwatering slow cooked meals that will help to restore your brain and overall health. Generally, this gluten-free cookbook will help you to further take hold of your birthright to live a long and healthy life.

Whatever you choose from this special collection of over 100 recipes, it's totally up to you. Just follow the instructions in this book and the different methods of preparing and cooking gluten-free will become surprisingly simple. In some cases, feel free to make your own gluten-free ingredient substitutions and tweak the recipes here and there based on your preferences or individual situations.

I have spent a lot of time to bring these recipes to perfection, but sometimes it's impossible to catch it all. So, if you see any glaring errors made in this book, please send me an email at shjensen@weightlosspeeps.com. I will be very grateful for your feedback.

Now, it's time to try your hand at creating healthy, easy and tasty gluten-free slow cooker meals using these specially created recipes.

Let's start cooking!

APPETIZERS

Sesame Almond Dip

This is a great recipe for a tasty dip. This dip will be nice as a spread for fresh fruit and vegetables.

Servings: 4
Prep Time: 15 minutes
Cooking Time: 4 hours

¼ cup Almonds, toasted and chopped

¼ cup Almond Milk

1 cup Almond Butter

½ teaspoon Curry Powder

2 tablespoons Sesame Seeds

Directions:

1. In a slow cooker, add all of the ingredients and mix well.

2. Set the slow cooker on low. Cover and cook for 4 hours.

Stuffed Jalapeño Peppers

This balanced spicy snack may be loved by everyone. In addition to being spicy, it is also healthy, thus a great dish for health conscious people.

Servings: 4
Prep Time: 20 minutes
Cooking Time: 4 hours

½ pound (226g) shredded cooked Chicken

¼ Green Bell Pepper, seeded and diced

¼ Yellow Bell Pepper, seeded and diced

1 small Onion, sliced

4 Jalapeño peppers, halved and seeded

Directions:

1. In a blender, add all of the ingredients, except for the jalapeño peppers, and pulse until mixed.

2. Stuff the pepper halves with the chicken mixture.

3. In a slow cooker, place the peppers in a single layer.

4. Set the slow cooker on low. Cover and cook for 4 hours.

Hot Mixed Nuts

This is a great nut recipe that is made with little or no fuss. These wonderfully crunchy snacks are often loved by everyone who tries them.

Servings: 4
Prep Time: 15 minutes
Cooking Time: 2 hours 15 minutes

---

2 teaspoons Extra Virgin Coconut Oil

½ teaspoon Smoked Paprika

½ teaspoon Cayenne Pepper

Flaked Sea Salt, to taste

Freshly Ground Black Pepper, to taste

½ cup Brazilian Nuts, shelled

½ cup Walnut Halves, chopped

½ cup Pecan Halves, chopped

Directions:

1. In a slow cooker, add all of the ingredients and mix well.

2. Set the slow cooker on high. Cover and cook for 15 minutes.

3. After 15 minutes stir the nuts and then set the slow cooker to low. Cover and cook for 2 hours.

Lemony Mushrooms

In this dish, the earthiness of fresh mushrooms is beautifully balanced by the lemon flavor of the broth. Serve this dish with a topping of freshly grated lemon zest.

Servings: 4
Prep Time: 15 minutes
Cooking Time: 12 hours

---

2 pounds (907g) fresh Mushrooms

2 cups Chicken Broth

1 tablespoon Fresh Lemon Juice

Flaked Sea Salt, to taste

Freshly Ground Black Pepper, to taste

1 teaspoon Dill Weed

3 tablespoons Coconut oil, Extra Virgin

Directions:

1. In a slow cooker mix together all of the ingredients.

2. Set the slow cooker on low. Cover and cook for 12 hours.

Mushy Liver Pate

This recipe is for a flavored beef liver and mushroom pate. It will be a great hit as a party snack, and will be wonderful with boiled eggs.

Servings: 4
Prep Time: 15 minutes
Cooking Time: 6 hours 5 minutes

---

1 tablespoon Extra Virgin Olive Oil

1 cup Fresh Mushrooms

1 medium Onion, chopped

3 Garlic Cloves, minced

½ cup Fresh Parsley

½ teaspoon Ground Nutmeg

Flaked Sea Salt, to taste

Freshly Ground Black Pepper, to taste

2 pounds (907g) Grass-Fed Beef Liver, cut into 2-inch pieces

Directions:

1. In a large skillet, heat the oil on a medium heat. Add all of the ingredients, except for the liver, and sauté for 5

minutes. Stir in the liver and transfer into a slow cooker.

2. Set the slow cooker on low. Cover and cook for 6 hours

3. Transfer the liver mixture into a large plate and allow to cool slightly.

4. In a blender add the mixture and pulse until smooth. Refrigerate to chill before serving.

Spiced Pumpkin Seeds

This is a delicious, crunchy and light snack for all. These spiced seeds are also great for topping soups.

Servings: 4
Prep Time: 10 minutes
Cooking Time: 4 hours

---

2 Organic Egg Whites

Flaked Sea Salt, to taste

Freshly Ground Black Pepper, to taste

½ teaspoon Cayenne Pepper

½ teaspoon Smoked Paprika

2 cups Pumpkin Seeds

Directions:

1. In a bowl, beat the egg whites until foamy. Add the salt, pepper, cayenne and paprika, and beat until mixed. Stir in the seeds.

2. Transfer the mixture into a slow cooker.

3. Set the slow cooker on low. Cover and cook for 4 hours.

Herbed Meatballs

This flavorful meatball dish is wonderfully slow cooked with fresh spices for a delightful treat. With a reasonably short preparation time, you may enjoy this dish as you as often as you want to.

Servings: 4
Prep Time: 20 minutes
Cooking Time: 8 hours

1¼ pounds (567g) Grass-Fed Lean Ground Beef

1 large Organic Egg, beaten

1 medium Onion, chopped finely

¼ cup Fresh Cilantro, chopped finely

2 tablespoons Fresh Thyme, chopped finely

2 tablespoons Fresh Oregano, chopped

¼ cup Almond Meal

Flaked Sea Salt, to taste

Freshly Ground Black Pepper, to taste

Directions:

1. In a large bowl, combine together all of the ingredients.

2. Make your desired sized meatballs from mixture. In a slow cooker, place the meatballs in a single row.

3. Set the slow cooker on low. Cover and cook for 8 hours.

Sweet & Spicy Mixed Nuts

This is an easy yet great snack idea to be served at any holiday party. These nuts have a light sweet and spicy taste with a wonderful crunch.

Servings: 4
Prep Time: 10 minutes
Cooking Time: 2 hours

---

3 tablespoons Coconut Oil, Extra Virgin

2 tablespoons Natural Stevia

½ teaspoon Ground Ginger

⅛ teaspoon Cayenne Pepper

¼ teaspoon Ground Cinnamon

⅛ teaspoon Ground Cloves

Flaked Sea Salt, to taste

Freshly Ground Black Pepper, to taste

¼ cup Hazelnuts, toasted and skin removed

½ cup Almonds, toasted

½ cup Walnut Halves, toasted

¼ cup Cashew nuts

Directions:

1. In a bowl, mix together the melted oil, stevia, ginger and spices.

2. In a slow cooker, place all of the nuts. Add the spice mixture, season with salt and pepper.

3. Set the slow cooker on low. Cover and cook for 1 hour.

4. Stir the nuts once and cover and cook for 1 hour more.

Spicy Chicken Kebobs

This recipe provides an easy way to prepare chicken kebobs. These kebobs will surely become a favorite snack for your whole family. Enjoy with your favorite dip.

Servings: 4
Prep Time: 15 minutes (plus time to marinate)
Cooking Time: 6 hours

---

2 pounds (907g) Grass-Fed skinless, boneless Chicken Breasts, sliced in half lengthwise

1 teaspoon Fresh Ginger, grated finely

½ teaspoon Garlic, minced

⅓ cup melted Extra Virgin Coconut Oil

¼ teaspoon Red Pepper Flakes, crushed

Flaked Sea Salt, to taste

Freshly Ground Black Pepper, to taste

Directions:

1. In a large bowl, add all of the ingredients and toss to coat well. Cover the bowl and refrigerate overnight. Mix the ingredients twice whilst refrigerating.

2. Thread the chicken pieces onto pre-soaked wooden skewers.

3. In a slow cooker, place the skewers in a single layer. Pour the marinade over the skewers.

4. Set the slow cooker on low. Cover and cook for 6 hours.

Nutty Stuffed Mushrooms

Stuffed mushrooms make a great appetizer or side dish to be served at a nice gathering. This dish also offers great nutrition and a wonderful taste.

Servings: 4
Prep Time: 15 minutes
Cooking Time: 2 hours 8 minutes

---

1 teaspoon Extra Virgin Coconut Oil

2 Garlic Cloves, sliced

½ cup Walnuts, chopped

Flaked Sea Salt, to taste

Freshly Ground Black Pepper, to taste

½ cup Fresh Spinach, chopped

½ cup White Onion, chopped

8 large Portobello Mushrooms, stems removed and chopped (do not chop the mushroom caps)

Directions:

1. In a skillet, heat the oil on a medium heat. Add the garlic, walnuts, salt and black pepper, and sauté for 4 to 5

minutes. Add the spinach, onion and chopped mushroom stems, and cook for 2 to 3 minutes.

2. Sprinkle the mushrooms caps with salt and black pepper. Evenly stuff the mushroom caps with the walnut mixture.

3. In a slow cooker, arrange the mushroom caps in a single row. Set the slow cooker on low. Cover and cook for 2 hours.

BREAKFAST

Mondie Meatloaf

This is one of the most convenient and easiest breakfast meatloaf recipes around. This dish is bursting with the flavors and aromas of the herbs used in the recipe. Garnish with fresh parsley leaves before serving.

Servings: 4
Prep Time: 15 minutes
Cooking Time: 3 hours

---

1 tablespoon Extra Virgin Olive Oil

1 cup Onion, diced

1 pound (454g) Grass-Fed Lean Ground Beef

1 Organic Egg, beaten

¼ cup Almond Flour

1 teaspoon Dried Oregano, crushed

1 teaspoon Dried Thyme, crushed

1 teaspoon Dried Rosemary, crushed

1 teaspoon Ground Fennel Seeds

½ teaspoon Smoked Paprika

1 teaspoon Red Pepper Flakes, crushed

Flaked Sea Salt, to taste

Freshly Ground Black Pepper, to taste

Directions:

1. In a pan, heat the oil on a medium heat. Add the onion and sauté for 4 to 5 minutes. Remove the pan from the heat and set to one side.

2. In a large bowl combine together the remaining ingredients. Stir in the cooked onion. Place the meat mixture in the center of a slow cooker, keeping a gap of about ½-inch from the sides of cooker. With your hands, shape the meat mixture in to a meatloaf form.

3. Set the slow cooker on low. Cover and cook for 3 hours.

Cheesy Chicken Casserole

This casserole is a delicious meal which is filled with the flavors of chicken and vegetables. The use of coconut milk gives a creamy touch to this dish. Garnish with freshly sliced scallions.

Servings: 4
Prep Time: 15 minutes
Cooking Time: 6-7 hours

---

1 teaspoon Extra virgin Olive Oil

1 pound (454g) diced Grass-Fed Boneless Chicken1 small Onion, sliced

1 large Green Bell Pepper, seeded and diced

1 large Yellow Bell Pepper, seeded and diced

1 large Red Bell Pepper, seeded and diced

1 medium Zucchini, diced

1 cup Mozzarella Cheese, shredded

10 Organic Eggs, beaten

1 cup Unsweetened Coconut Milk

Flaked Sea Salt, to taste

Freshly Ground Black Pepper, to taste

Pinch of Red Pepper Flakes, crushed

Directions:

1. In a skillet, heat the oil on a medium heat. Add the chicken and cook for 4 to 5 minutes. Set aside the chicken on a plate. In a bowl, mix together all the vegetables. In another bowl combine together the eggs, coconut milk, salt, black pepper and red pepper flakes.

2. Grease a slow cooker. Place half of the chicken in the bottom of the cooker. Place half of the onion over the chicken. Spread half of the vegetables over the onion and sprinkle with half of the cheese. Repeat the process to create another layer.

3. Pour the beaten egg mixture on top.

4. Set the slow cooker on low. Cover and cook for 4 to 5 hours.

Beef Butternut Casserole

With this recipe, a little bit of preparation is rewarded by producing a warm and tasty breakfast casserole ready for when you get out of bed in the morning. Top with fresh cilantro leaves.

Servings: 4
Prep Time: 15 minutes
Cooking Time: 8 -10 hours

---

1 teaspoon Extra Virgin Coconut Oil

1 small Onion, chopped

1 pound (454g) Grass-Fed Lean Ground Beef

Flaked Sea Salt, to taste

Freshly Ground Black Pepper, to taste

1 cup Unsweetened Almond Milk

10 Organic Eggs

1 large peeled, seeded and chopped Summer Squash

Directions:

1. In a pan, heat the oil on a medium heat. Add the onion and sauté for 4 to 5 minutes. Add the beef and sprinkle with salt and black pepper before cooking for 4 to 5

minutes.

2. In a bowl beat together the almond milk and eggs.

3. Grease a slow cooker. Place the beef mixture and chopped squash into the slow cooker. Pour in the egg mixture and mix well.

4. Set the slow cooker on low. Cover and cook overnight or for 8 to 10 hours.

Chicken Zucchini Frittata

This is a hearty and delicious breakfast frittata. Each of the ingredients in this recipe brings a wonderful flavor to this dish. Garnish with sliced scallion.

Servings: 4
Prep Time: 15 minutes
Cooking Time: 6-8 hours

---

1 teaspoon Extra Virgin Coconut Oil

1 small yellow Onion, chopped

1 pound (454g) Grass-Fed Ground Chicken

8 Organic Eggs, beaten

2 large Zucchinis, peeled, seeded and chopped

1 teaspoon Dried Thyme, crushed

1 teaspoon Dried Oregano, crushed

Flaked Sea Salt, to taste

Freshly Ground Black Pepper, to taste

Directions:

1. Grease a slow cooker. Place all of the ingredients in the cooker and mix well.

2. Set the slow cooker on low. Cover and cook for 6 to 8 hours.

Beef & Kale Quiche

This quiche is absolutely delicious. The flavor combination of beef, kale, scallions and eggs complement each other nicely. Serve with avocado slices.

Servings: 4
Prep Time: 15 minutes
Cooking Time: 6 -7 hours

---

1 tablespoon Extra Virgin Olive Oil

1 pound (454g) Grass-Fed Lean Ground Beef

2 teaspoons Garlic, minced

5 cups Kale, trimmed and chopped roughly

2 cups Scallions, chopped

8 Organic Eggs, beaten

Directions:

1. In a pan, heat ½ tablespoon of the oil on a medium heat. Add the beef and cook for 4 to 5 minutes. Transfer the beef onto a plate. In the same pan, heat the remaining oil on a medium heat. Add the garlic, kale and scallion, and sauté for 4 to 5 minutes. Remove from the heat.

2. In a bowl beat together the milk and eggs.

3. Place the beef and vegetable mixture into a slow cooker. Pour over the beaten eggs and stir to mix well.

4. Set the slow cooker to low. Cover and cook for 6 to 7 hours.

Vegetable & Chicken Casserole

This is a healthy and delicious recipe that is perfect either for breakfast, lunch or maybe even dinner. The use of turnips in this dish provides a classic taste. Serve with the slices of avocado.

Servings: 4
Prep Time: 15 minutes
Cooking Time: 8 -10 hours

---

1 ½ tablespoons Extra Virgin Olive Oil

1 pound (454g) Grass-Fed Skinless, Boneless Chicken, cut into bite sized pieces

1 Green Bell Pepper, seeded and diced

1 Red Onion, diced

2 Garlic Cloves, minced

3 large Turnips, peeled and grated

Pinch of Red Pepper Flakes, crushed

1 cup Unsweetened Almond Milk

12 Organic Eggs

1 teaspoon Dried Dill Weed, crushed

Flaked Sea Salt, to taste

Freshly Ground Black Pepper, to taste

Directions:

1. In a pan, heat ½ tablespoon of oil on a medium heat. Add the chicken and cook for 4 to 5 minutes. Transfer the chicken onto a plate. In the same pan, heat the remaining oil on a medium heat. Add the bell pepper, onion and garlic and sauté for 4 to 5 minutes. Stir in the chicken and remove from the heat.

2. In a bowl, mix together the grated turnip and red pepper flakes. In another bowl beat together the milk, eggs, dill, salt and black pepper.

3. Grease a slow cooker. Place ⅓ of the turnip mixture into the slow cooker. Then place ⅓ of the chicken mixture on top. Top with ⅓ of the egg mixture. Repeat the layers twice more.

4. Set the slow cooker on low. Cover and cook for 8 to 10 hours.

Crunchy Apple Pudding

This breakfast pudding with its crunchy cinnamon topping is one of those family favorites. Serve as a warm breakfast with the topping of nuts of your choice.

Servings: 4
Prep Time: 20 minutes
Cooking Time: 4 hours, plus 1 hour to rest.

For Pudding:

½ cup Water

1 cup Unsweetened Almond Milk

1 tablespoon Arrowroot Powder

½ cup Chia Seeds

1 teaspoon Ground Cinnamon

Pinch of Flaked Sea Salt

3 large Apples, cored and sliced

For Topping:

¼ cup blanched Almond Flour

1 tablespoon Natural Stevia

½ teaspoon Ground Cinnamon

2 tablespoons Coconut, unsweetened and shredded

2 tablespoons Unsweetened Applesauce

½ teaspoon Vanilla Extract

Directions:

1. In a slow cooker, mix together all of the pudding ingredients, except for the apple. Arrange the apple slices over the milk mixture.

2. In a bowl, mix together all of the topping ingredients. Sprinkle the topping mixture over the apple slices.

3. Set the slow cooker on low. Cover and cook for 4 hours.

4. After 4 hours turn off the heat. Leave the dish in the covered pan for at least a further hour to rest. Top with crushed nuts before serving.

Berry Crumble

This is a delicious breakfast for the whole family. The medley of berries with a crumble topping makes a wonderfully delicious breakfast. Sprinkle with ground cinnamon.

Servings: 4
Prep Time: 20 minutes
Cooking Time: 2 hours

---

4 cups mixed Fresh Berries (for example Raspberries, Blackberries and Strawberries)

3 tablespoons Almond Butter, melted and divided

1 cup Almond Flour

½ tablespoon Natural Stevia

Directions:

1. Arrange the berries on the base of a slow cooker and drizzle with 1 tablespoon of the butter.

2. In a bowl add the remaining butter, flour and stevia, and mix until a crumble forms.

3. Evenly cover the berries with the crumble mixture.

4. Set the slow cooker on low. Cover and cook for 2 hours.

Spiced Fruit Plate

This is an elegant and perfect breakfast that even the kids may enjoy. The spices used in this recipe provide a wonderful balance to the peaches and cranberries.

Servings: 4
Prep Time: 20 minutes
Cooking Time: 4 hours

---

4 Pears, peeled and cored

¼ teaspoon Ground Nutmeg

¼ teaspoon Ground Cinnamon

1 tablespoon Extra Virgin Olive Oil

½ teaspoon Vanilla Extract

1 cup Fresh Cranberries

Directions:

1. Arrange the pears upright in a slow cooker. Sprinkle with the nutmeg and cinnamon.

2. In a bowl combine together the oil and vanilla. Pour the oil mixture over the pears. Top with the cranberries.

3. Set the slow cooker on low. Cover and cook for 4 hours.

Nuts & Seeds Granola

This is a very healthy breakfast for the whole family. This granola is a mixture of nuts and seeds coated in egg whites and spices. Top with fresh berries before serving.

Servings: 4
Prep Time: 20 minutes
Cooking Time: 2 hours

---

2 large Organic Egg Whites

1 tablespoon Natural Stevia

2 teaspoons Vanilla Extract

½ teaspoon Ground Allspice

½ teaspoon Ground Ginger

2 teaspoons Ground Cinnamon

½ cup Almonds, chopped

½ cup Walnuts, chopped

½ cup Pecans, chopped

½ cup Pumpkin Seeds, toasted

1 tablespoon Extra Virgin Coconut Oil

Directions:

1. In a bowl combine together the egg whites, stevia, vanilla and spices, and stir in the nuts.

2. Grease a slow cooker. Pour the nut mixture into the prepared cooker and drizzle with melted coconut oil.

3. Set the slow cooker on high. Cook for 2 to 3 hours, stirring after every 20 minutes.

CHICKEN RECIPES

Easgo Chicken Drumsticks

This is an easy, slow cooked chicken dish, made with little or no fuss. Serve with a drizzling of fresh lemon juice.

Servings: 4
Prep Time: 10 minutes
Cooking Time: 4 hours, 10 minutes

---

8 Grass-Fed skinless Chicken Drumsticks

½ teaspoon Red Pepper Flakes, crushed

Flaked Sea Salt, to taste

Freshly Ground Black Pepper, to taste

Directions:

1. Using a sharp knife, make deep cuts into the chicken drumsticks. Sprinkle the drumsticks generously with salt, red pepper flakes and black pepper.

2. Grease a slow cooker. Arrange the drumsticks in the

3. prepared cooker.

4. Set the slow cooker on low. Cover and cook for 3 to 4 hours.

5. Preheat the grill to a medium-high heat. Grease the grill grate. Cook the drumsticks, turning once, for a further 10 minutes.

Creamy Chicken Curry

These chicken thighs and bell peppers are cooked in a wonder blend of coconut milk, cashew butter, curry powder and fresh herbs. This recipe makes a delicious chicken dish. Serve with fresh lime slices.

Servings: 4
Prep Time: 20 minutes
Cooking Time: 5hours, 30 minutes

---

2 cups Coconut Milk, unsweetened

2 tablespoons Cashew Butter

2 teaspoons Curry Powder

½ teaspoon Red Pepper Flakes, crushed

Flaked Sea Salt, to taste

4 Grass-Fed skinless, boneless Chicken Thighs

1 Green Bell Pepper, seeded and sliced

1 Red Bell Pepper, seeded and sliced

½ medium Yellow Onion, sliced

1 Celery Stalk, sliced

2 tablespoons Fresh Thyme, chopped

2 tablespoons Fresh Basil, chopped

Directions:

1. In a bowl, mix together the coconut milk, butter, curry powder, red pepper flakes and salt. Pour the milk mixture in a slow cooker.

2. In the slow cooker, mix together the remaining ingredients.

3. Set the slow cooker on low. Cover and cook for 5½ hours.

Roasted Apple Chicken

This roasted chicken has a hint of lime which tastes fabulous.
Serve this tasty chicken on a bed of fresh lettuce leaves.

Servings: 4
Prep Time: 15 minutes
Cooking Time: 6 hours

---

1 tablespoon Lime Zest, freshly grated

2 Garlic Cloves, minced

¼ teaspoon Ground All Spice

Flaked Sea Salt, to taste

Freshly Ground Black Pepper, to taste

1 (3-pound) (1361g) Grass-Fed Whole Roasting Chicken

1 tablespoon Extra Virgin Olive Oil

1 Lime, sliced

1 small Apple, cored and chopped

Directions:

1. Mix together the lime zest, garlic, all spice, salt and black pepper. Rub the chicken cavity with salt and black pepper

generously.

2. Evenly coat the chicken with oil and rub the chicken with the garlic mixture.

3. Fill the cavity of the chicken with lime and apple pieces. With kitchen string, tie the legs of chicken. Arrange the chicken in a slow cooker.

4. Set the slow cooker on low. Cover and cook for about 6 hours.

Spiced Creamy Chicken

This is a very simple, nutritious yet flavorful chicken dish. The combination of the ingredients creates a unique flavor. Top with toasted and chopped almonds before serving.

Servings: 4
Prep Time: 15 minutes
Cooking Time: 6 hours, 5 minutes

---

1 tablespoon Extra Virgin Olive Oil

4 Grass-Fed skinless, boneless Chicken Thighs

1 large Onion, sliced

1 tablespoon Fresh Ginger, minced

6 Garlic Cloves, minced

1 Green Chili, minced

1½ cups Fresh Cilantro, chopped

1 tablespoon Fresh Mint, chopped

¾ teaspoon Ground Cilantro

½ teaspoon Ground Cumin

Pinch of Cayenne Pepper

Flaked Sea Salt, to taste

Freshly Ground Black Pepper, to taste

1¾ cups Coconut Milk, unsweetened

Directions:

1. In a skillet, heat the oil on a medium-high heat. Cook the chicken for 4 to 5 minutes, or until golden brown. Remove from the heat.

2. In a slow cooker, mix together the remaining ingredients. Place the chicken thighs in the slow cooker and lightly press them into the milk mixture.

3. Set the slow cooker on low. Cover and cook for 5½ to 6 hours.

Hot Chicken Zucchini

This is a nutritional and a great tasting recipe for chicken combined with zucchini. Enjoy this dish with a garnishing of chopped cashews.

Servings: 4
Prep Time: 15 minutes
Cooking Time: 4 hours, 5 minutes

---

1 teaspoon Extra Virgin Olive Oil

4 Grass-Fed skinless, boneless Chicken Breasts

Flaked Sea Salt, to taste

Freshly Ground Black Pepper, to taste

1 cup Homemade Low-sodium Chicken Broth

½ cup Coconut Milk, unsweetened

1 tablespoon Cashew Butter

½ teaspoon Red Pepper Flakes, crushed

½ teaspoon Cayenne Pepper

2 Garlic Cloves, minced

½ teaspoon Fresh Ginger, minced

2 Large Zucchinis, sliced thinly

1 Bunch Scallions, sliced

Directions:

1. In a skillet, heat the oil on a medium-high heat. Sprinkle the chicken with salt and black pepper and cook until golden brown, or for 4 to 5 minutes. Remove the skillet from the heat.

2. In a bowl, add the broth, coconut milk, butter, red pepper flakes, cayenne pepper, salt and black pepper, and beat until combined. Transfer the broth mixture into a slow cooker.

3. Add the chicken, garlic and ginger, and mix well. Top with the zucchini and scallions.

4. Set the slow cooker on low. Cover and cook for 3½ to 4 hours.

Garlic Pepper Chicken

The almond butter and lemon juice used in this recipe adds a wonderful flavor to the chicken. Serve this chicken with steamed broccoli.

Servings: 4
Prep Time: 10 minutes
Cooking Time: 8 hours

---

1 pound (454g) Grass-Fed boneless, skinless Chicken Breasts

⅓ cup Almond Butter

1 teaspoon Garlic, minced

½ teaspoon Fresh Ginger, minced

2 tablespoons Fresh Lemon juice

¾ cup Homemade Low-sodium Chicken Broth

½ teaspoon Red Pepper Flakes, crushed

Flaked Sea Salt, to taste

Freshly Ground Black Pepper, to taste

Directions:

1. Grease a slow cooker. Mix together all of the ingredients

in the prepared slow cooker.

2. Set the slow cooker on low. Cover and cook for 6 to 8 hours.

Chocolaty Chicken Frita

This is a hearty and flavorful chicken meal. The blend of dark chocolate and spices with almond butter adds a richness and amazing flavors to the chicken. Serve with avocado slices.

Servings: 4
Prep Time: 15 minutes
Cooking Time: 6 hours, 11 minutes

---

1 tablespoon Extra Virgin Olive Oil

1½ pounds (680g) Grass-fed skinless Chicken Legs

Flaked Sea Salt, to taste

Freshly Ground Black Pepper, to taste

1 small Onion, chopped

1 teaspoon Garlic, minced

½ teaspoon Fresh Ginger, minced

5-6 Fresh, peeled, seeded and chopped Roma Tomatoes

2 Serrano Chiles, seeded and chopped

3 tablespoons Almond Butter

2-ounces (56g) 70% Dark Chocolate

1 teaspoon Ground Cumin

½ teaspoon Cayenne Pepper

Directions:

1. In a skillet, heat the oil on a medium-high heat. Sprinkle the chicken with salt and black pepper and cook until golden brown, or for 4 to 5 minutes. Transfer the chicken into a slow cooker.

2. In the same skillet, add the onion and sauté for 4 to 5 minutes. Add the garlic and ginger and sauté for a further minute. Transfer the onion mixture into a slow cooker. Mix in the remaining ingredients.

3. Set the slow cooker on low. Cover and cook for about 4 to 6 hours.

Tangy Chicken Delight

This is a delicious and family friendly recipe which may satisfy everyone's taste buds. Serve with a topping of sliced scallions.

Servings: 4
Prep Time: 15 minutes (plus time to marinate)
Cooking Time: 6 hours, 11 minutes

---

1 tablespoon Extra Virgin Olive Oil

3 pounds (1361g) Grass-fed skinless Chicken Wings

½ teaspoon Cayenne Pepper

½ teaspoon Smoked Paprika

1 teaspoon Ground Cumin

Flaked Sea Salt, to taste

Freshly Ground White Pepper, to taste

2 tablespoons Fresh Lime juice

2 tablespoons Fresh Lemon juice

Directions:

1. In a skillet, heat the oil on a medium-high heat. Add the

chicken wings and sprinkle with salt and black pepper. Cook for 4 to 5 minutes, or until golden brown. Transfer the chicken into a large bowl.

2. In a bowl, mix together all of the spices. Generously sprinkle the chicken with the spice mixture. Add the remaining ingredients and toss to coat well. Refrigerate overnight in a covered dish.

3. Transfer the chicken wings, with marinade, into a slow cooker.

4. Set the slow cooker on low. Cover and cook for about 4 hours.

Spicy Chicken with Cauliflower

This chicken dish is delicious and nice in a spicy way. Warm spices and creamy coconut milk add a great flavor and moisture to the chicken *and cauliflower. Garnish with freshly grated lime zest.*

Servings: 4
Prep Time: 15 minutes
Cooking Time: 6 hours, 12 minutes

¼ teaspoon Cayenne Pepper

½ teaspoon Ground Turmeric

½ teaspoon Ground Cilantro

½ teaspoon Ground Cumin

Pinch of Ground Cloves

Flaked Sea Salt, to taste

Freshly Ground Black Pepper, to taste

1 pound (454g) Grass-fed boneless, skinless Chicken Breasts

2 tablespoons Extra Virgin Coconut Oil

1 small Onion, chopped

2 Garlic Cloves, minced

½ teaspoon Fresh Ginger, minced

1 Fresh Green Chili, chopped

1 Cauliflower Head, cut into florets

1 cup Coconut Milk, unsweetened

Directions:

1. In a bowl, mix together all of the spices. Add the chicken and generously coat with the spice mixture. Set to one side for 10 minutes.

2. In a skillet, heat 1 tablespoon of the oil on a medium heat. Add the chicken and cook until golden brown, or for 4 to 5 minutes. Remove the chicken onto a plate.

3. In the same skillet, heat the remaining oil on a medium heat. Add the onion and sauté for 4 to 5 minutes. Add the garlic and ginger, and sauté for a further 2 minutes. Transfer the onion mixture into a slow cooker. Place the cauliflower and green chili in the slow cooker. Top with the chicken. Pour the coconut milk over chicken.

4. Set the slow cooker on low. Cover and cook for about 6 hours.

Chicken Jicama

This is an easy and tasty meal with a kick of spice. The jicama combines well with the ground chicken and spices. Serve with fresh greens.

Servings: 4
Prep Time: 15 minutes
Cooking Time: 6 hours, 10 minutes

---

1 tablespoon Extra Virgin Olive Oil

1 pound (454g) Grass-fed Lean Ground Chicken

2 Onions, chopped

4 Garlic Cloves, minced

½ teaspoon Fresh Ginger, minced

½ cup Homemade Low-sodium Chicken Broth

2 tablespoons Fresh Lemon juice

½ cup Jicama, peeled and chopped

¼ teaspoon Cayenne Pepper

¼ teaspoon Red Pepper Flakes, crushed

½ teaspoon Ground Cumin

Flaked Sea Salt, to taste

Freshly Ground Black Pepper, to taste

2 tablespoons Scallions, sliced thinly

Directions:

1. In a skillet, heat the oil on a medium-high heat. Add the ground chicken and sprinkle with salt and black pepper. Cook for 4 to 5 minutes, or until golden brown. Transfer the chicken into a slow cooker.

2. Add the remaining ingredients and mix well.

3. Set the slow cooker on low. Cover and cook for 6 to 8 hours.

4. Uncover and stir in the scallions. Cook, uncovered, for about 5 minutes more.

MEAT RECIPES

Lemony Beef Roast

This is a refreshing tangy twist to a traditional beef roast. This dish is enhanced by the use of fresh lemon juice, green chilies and thyme. Serve with fresh lemon slices.

Servings: 4
Prep Time: 10 minutes
Cooking Time: 8 hours

---

2 pounds (907g) Grass-Fed Beef Roast

¼ cup Fresh Lemon juice

½ cup Homemade Low-sodium Beef Broth

2-3 Garlic Cloves, minced

½ cup Fresh Green Chilies, seeded and chopped

1 teaspoon Dried Thyme, crushed

2 teaspoons Ground Cumin

Flaked Sea Salt, to taste

Directions:

1. Place the beef into a slow cooker. In a bowl, mix together all of the remaining ingredients. Pour the mixture over the beef.

2. Set the slow cooker on low. Cover and cook for 6 to 8 hours.

Beef with Mushrooms

This is an awesome and flavorful recipe. The combination of mushrooms, celery *and onions complement the beef perfectly. Garnish with chopped fresh scallions.*

Servings: 4
Prep Time: 10 minutes
Cooking Time: 8 hours, 45 minutes

2 pounds (907g) Grass-Fed Beef Shoulder

1 cup Homemade Low-sodium Beef Broth

1 small Onion, sliced

2 Celery Stalks, sliced

2 Garlic Cloves, minced

Flaked Sea Salt, to taste

Freshly Ground Black Pepper, to taste

1 ¼ cups Fresh Mushrooms, halved

Directions:

1. Mix together all of the ingredients, except for the mushrooms, into a slow cooker.

2. Set the cooker on low. Cover and cook for 6 to 8 hours.

3. Open the slow cooker. Stir in the mushrooms. Cover and cook for a further 45 minutes.

Peppered Ground Beef

This is a classic chili recipe with a mixture of beef, bell peppers, tomatoes, serrano and seasoning. This chili may win over the pickiest of eaters. Garnish with freshly chopped herbs.

Servings: 4
Prep Time: 20 minutes
Cooking Time: 5 hours, 10 minutes

---

1 tablespoon Extra Virgin Olive Oil

1 small Onion, chopped

4 Garlic Cloves, minced

1 pound (454g) Grass-Fed Lean Ground Beef

4 Stalks Celery, chopped

1 Green Bell Pepper, seeded and chopped

1 Red Bell Pepper, seeded and chopped

1 Yellow Bell Pepper, seeded and chopped

2½ cups Fresh Tomatoes, chopped finely

1 Serrano Chili, chopped

1½ teaspoons Ground Cumin

2 teaspoons Chili Powder

1 teaspoon Smoked Paprika

½ teaspoon Dried Oregano, crushed

½ teaspoon Dried Thyme, crushed

Flaked Sea Salt, to taste

Directions:

1. In a skillet, heat the oil on a medium heat. Sauté the onion and garlic for 4 to 5 minutes. Add the beef and cook for 4 to 5 minutes. Transfer the beef mixture into a slow cooker.

2. Add all of the remaining ingredients and mix.

3. Set the slow cooker on low. Cover and cook for 4 to 5 hours.

Chili Beef Steak

This recipe makes one of the most tender and spicy shredded beef dishes you will ever taste. This delicious beef dish is also really simple to prepare. Serve on a bed of cabbage leaves.

Servings: 4
Prep Time: 10 minutes
Cooking Time: 10 hours

1½ pounds (680g) Grass-Fed Sirloin Steak

½ cup Homemade Low-sodium Beef Broth

1 large Onion, sliced

¼ teaspoon Smoked Paprika

¼ teaspoon Chili Powder

Freshly Ground White Pepper, to taste

Flaked Sea Salt, to taste

Freshly Ground Black Pepper, to taste

Directions:

1. Mix together all of the ingredients in a slow cooker.

2. Set the slow cooker on low. Cover and cook for 8 to 10 hours.

3. Shred the meat before serving.

Beef Broccoli

This authentic recipe is prepared with a mild spicy touch. This beef with broccoli dish is great for lunch or as a dinner. Garnish with freshly grated lemon zest.

Servings: 4
Prep Time: 15 minutes
Cooking Time: 6 hours, 21 minutes

---

1 tablespoon Extra Virgin Olive Oil

2 Garlic Cloves, minced

1 pound (454g) Grass-Fed Flank Steak, cubed

½ cup Homemade Low-sodium Beef Broth

1 tablespoon Fresh Lemon juice

½ teaspoon Smoked Paprika

½ teaspoon Red Pepper Flakes that are crushed

Flaked Sea Salt, to taste

Freshly Ground Black Pepper, to taste

1 tablespoon Fresh Ginger, grated

2 cups Broccoli, chopped

Directions:

1. In a skillet, heat the oil on a medium-high heat and sauté the garlic for 1 minute. Add the beef and cook for 4 to 5 minutes per side. Transfer the beef mixture into a slow cooker.

2. Add the remaining ingredients, except for the broccoli, and mix.

3. Set the slow cooker on low. Cover and cook for 4 to 5½ hours.

4. Open the slow cooker and stir in the broccoli. Cook, covered, for 30 to 45 minutes.

Garlicky Short Ribs

These short ribs are moist and tender once cooked. Your family and friends will love to eat these ribs time and again. Serve with a side dish of steamed green beans.

Servings: 4
Prep Time: 10 minutes
Cooking Time: 6 hours, 4 minutes

---

1 tablespoon Extra Virgin Coconut Oil

2 pounds (907g) Grass-Fed Beef Short Ribs

6 Garlic Cloves, mashed

1 tablespoon Smoked Paprika

1 teaspoon Red Pepper Flakes, crushed

Flaked Sea Salt, to taste

Freshly Ground Black Pepper, to taste

¾ cup Homemade Low-sodium Beef Broth

Directions:

1. In a skillet, heat the oil on a medium-high heat. Add the ribs and cook for 2 minutes per side. Transfer the ribs into a slow cooker.

2. Top the ribs with the garlic.

3. In a bowl, mix together the remaining ingredients. Pour the mixture over the beef.

4. Set the slow cooker on low. Cover and cook for 5 to 6 hours.

Mustard Glazed Beef

This is one of the gem recipes for short ribs. The secret ingredient to these succulent ribs is Dijon mustard, this adds a rich flavoring. Serve with grilled broccoli.

Servings: 4
Prep Time: 10 minutes
Cooking Time: 8 hours, 4 minutes

---

1 tablespoon Extra Virgin Olive Oil

2 pounds (907g) Grass-Fed Beef Short Ribs

Flaked Sea Salt, to taste

Freshly Ground Black Pepper, to taste

1 tablespoon Dijon Mustard

2 tablespoons Fresh Lemon Juice

½ cup Homemade Low-sodium Beef Broth

Directions:

1. In a skillet, heat the oil on a medium-high heat. Add the ribs and sprinkle with salt and black pepper. Cook for 2 minutes per side. Transfer the ribs into a slow cooker.

2. In a bowl, add the remaining ingredients and beat until combined. Pour the mustard mixture over the beef.

3. Set the slow cooker on low. Cover and cook for about 8 hours.

Zesty Beef Zucchini

This is a meat recipe that has healthy proteins and the powerful nutritional value of zucchinis. This recipe makes a great dish for dinner. Top with sliced scallion.

Servings: 4
Prep Time: 15 minutes
Cooking Time: 8 hours

½ cup Homemade Low-sodium Beef Broth

1 tablespoon Arrowroot Powder

1½ pounds (680g) Grass-Fed Eye of Round Roast

1 Plum Tomato, chopped

1 medium Zucchini, chopped

1 small Onion, sliced

1 Garlic Clove, minced

2 tablespoons Fresh Lemon Juice

1 tablespoon Fresh Oregano, chopped

Flaked Sea Salt, to taste

Freshly Ground Black Pepper, to taste

Directions:

1. In a bowl, mix together the broth and arrowroot powder.

2. In a slow cooker, mix together the remaining ingredients. Pour the broth over the meat.

3. Set the slow cooker on low. Cover and cook for 6 to 8 hours.

Curried Beef Squash

This is a delicious and a great tasting beef curry which is ideal for a chilly evening. The lemongrass and lime leaves lighten the flavor of the meat nicely. Garnish with freshly grated lime zest.

Servings: 4
Prep Time: 20 minutes
Cooking Time: 8 hours, 5 minutes

1 tablespoon Extra Virgin Olive Oil

1½ pounds (680g) Grass-Fed boneless Beef, sliced into ¼-inch thickness

1½ cups unsweetened Coconut Milk

2 small Yellow Squash, sliced

2 Garlic Cloves, minced

1 tablespoon Fresh Ginger, grated

2 Fresh Lime Leaves

1 Stalk Lemon Grass, sliced

2 tablespoons Curry Powder

1 teaspoon Chili Powder

1 teaspoon Ground Cumin

1 teaspoon Ground Cilantro

Flaked Sea Salt, to taste

Freshly Ground Black Pepper, to taste

Directions:

1. In a skillet, heat the oil on a medium-high heat. Add the beef and cook for 4 to 5 minutes. Transfer the beef into a slow cooker.

2. Add the remaining ingredients and mix.

3. Set the slow cooker on low. Cover and cook for 6 to 8 hours.

Meatballs with Tomato Sauce

This is one of the best homemade, comforting and delicious dishes.
Your whole family, especially kids, will love this. Serve with a
garnishing of fresh cilantro leaves.

Servings: 4
Prep Time: 20 minutes
Cooking Time: 6 hours, 5 minutes

1½ pounds (680g) Grass-Fed Lean Ground Beef

1 medium Onion, chopped

8 Garlic Cloves, minced and divided

2 tablespoons Fresh Cilantro, chopped finely

1 tablespoon Fresh Mint, chopped finely

¼ cup Almond Meal

2 Organic Medium Eggs, beaten

Flaked Sea Salt, to taste

Freshly Ground Black Pepper, to taste

1 tablespoon Extra Virgin Olive Oil

¾ cup Homemade Tomato Paste

2 cups Tomatoes, chopped finely

½ cup Fresh Thyme, chopped finely

Directions:

1. In a large bowl, mix together the beef, onion, 4 garlic cloves, cilantro, mint, almond meal, eggs, salt and black pepper. Form the mixture into balls. In a skillet, heat the oil on a medium heat. Add the balls and cook for 4 to 5 minutes, or until browned. Transfer the balls into a slow cooker.

2. In another large bowl, mix the remaining garlic with the tomato paste, chopped tomatoes and thyme. Pour the tomato mixture over the meatballs.

3. Set the slow cooker on low. Cover and cook for 4 to 6 hours.

Lamb Shoulder Curry

This recipe has a wonderful depth of flavor. The combination of coconut milk and spices gives a delicious taste to the beef. Garnish with fresh basil leaves.

Servings: 4
Prep Time: 10 minutes
Cooking Time: 5 hours

---

1 pound (454g) Grass-Fed Lamb Shoulder (bone-in), cut into pieces

1¼ cups unsweetened Coconut Milk

2 tablespoons Fresh Lime juice

1 small Onion, chopped

1 teaspoon Fresh Ginger, grated

2 Garlic Cloves, minced

1 teaspoon Curry Powder

⅛ teaspoon Chili Powder

¼ teaspoon ground Turmeric

1 teaspoon Ground Cumin

1 teaspoon Ground Cilantro

⅛ teaspoon Ground Cinnamon

⅛ teaspoon Ground Cloves

Flaked Sea Salt, to taste

Directions:

1. Place the lamb pieced into a slow cooker.

2. In a bowl, mix together the remaining ingredients. Pour the coconut milk mixture over the lamb and mix.

3. Set the slow cooker on low. Cover and cook for about 5 hours.

Herbed Leg of Lamb

This amazing recipe is perfect for special occasions. You are guaranteed to enjoy this dish every time you serve it. Serve with roasted turnips.

Servings: 4
Prep Time: 10 minutes (Plus time to marinate)
Cooking Time: 3 hours, 30 minutes

½ cup Fresh Rosemary, minced

¼ cup Fresh Thyme, minced

¼ cup Fresh Oregano, minced

2 Garlic Cloves, minced

1 tablespoon Plain Mustard

1 teaspoon Smoked Paprika

1 teaspoon Red Pepper Flakes, crushed

Flaked Sea Salt, to taste

Freshly Ground Black Pepper, to taste

2½ pounds (1134g) Grass-Fed Leg of Lamb (bone-in)

Directions:

1. In a large bowl, mix together all of the ingredients, except for the lamb. Generously rub the leg of lamb with the herb mixture. Cover and refrigerate to marinate for 6 to 8 hours.

2. Remove the lamb from the refrigerator and sit at room temperature for about 30 minutes.

3. Place the leg of lamb in a slow cooker.

4. Set the slow cooker on low. Cover and cook for 2½ to 3½ hours.

Lamb Shanks with Tomato Sauce

This is the ultimate comfort food dish for supper for the whole family. These lamb shanks are really tender and full of flavor. Serve with fresh greens.

Servings: 4
Prep Time: 15 minutes
Cooking Time: 6 hours, 5 minutes

1½ tablespoons Coconut Oil, Extra Virgin

4 Grass-Fed Lamb Shanks, trimmed

Flaked Sea Salt, to taste

Freshly Ground Black Pepper, to taste

1 large White Onion, chopped

3 Garlic Cloves, minced

3 Celery Stalks, chopped

2 tablespoons Homemade Tomato Paste

1½ cups Tomatoes, peeled, seeded and chopped finely

1 tablespoon Fresh Oregano, minced

1 Bay Leaf

2½ cups Homemade Low-sodium Chicken Broth

Directions:

1. In a skillet, heat the oil on a medium-high heat. Add the lamb shanks and cook for 4 to 5 minutes. Transfer the shanks into a slow cooker. Add the remaining ingredients and mix.

2. Set the slow cooker on high. Cover and cook for about 6 hours.

3. Transfer the shanks onto a serving plate. Discard the bay leaf and, with a blender, blend the tomato mixture until a puree forms.

4. Top the shanks with the tomato puree before serving.

Roasted Lamb Chops

These delicious and flavorful roasted lamb chops *make a perfect midweek supper. The aroma of these chops is irresistible. Serve with fresh greens.*

Servings: 4
Prep Time: 10 minutes
Cooking Time: 6 hours

½ teaspoon Dried Oregano, crushed

½ teaspoon Dried Thyme, crushed

Flaked Sea Salt, to taste

Freshly Ground Black Pepper, to taste

8 Grass-Fed Lamb Loin Chops

1 medium Onion, sliced

3 Garlic Cloves, minced

Directions:

1. In a large bowl, mix together the herbs, salt and black pepper. Generously rub the lamb chops with the herb mixture.

2. Place the onions into a slow cooker. Arrange the chops over the onion and top with the garlic.

3. Set the slow cooker on low. Cover and cook for 4 to 6 hours.

Celery Loin Chops

These lamb chops are fantastic for a Sunday night dinner. This dish is truly delicious even though it is being made from simple ingredients. Garnish with sliced scallion.

Servings: 4
Prep Time: 15 minutes
Cooking Time: 7 hours, 5 minutes

1½ tablespoons Coconut Oil, Extra Virgin

8 Grass-Fed Lamb Loin Chops

1⅓ cups Homemade Low-sodium Chicken Broth

2 tablespoons Homemade Tomato Paste

4 Celery Ribs, chopped

1 Garlic Clove, minced

1½ cups Tomatoes, peeled, seeded and chopped finely

1 teaspoon Red Pepper Flakes, crushed

Flaked Sea Salt, to taste

Freshly Ground Black Pepper, to taste

Directions:

1. In a skillet, heat the oil on a medium-high heat. Add the lamb chops and cook for 4 to 5 minutes. Transfer the chops into a slow cooker.

2. In the same skillet, add the remaining ingredients and bring to the boil. Pour the broth mixture over the chops.

3. Set the slow cooker on low. Cover and cook for 5to 7 hours.

Olives & Garlic Lamb

This rich and tasty dish is bursting with flavor. The use of lamb and olives with dried herbs make a perfect combination. Garnish with freshly grated lime zest.

Servings: 4
Prep Time: 15 minutes
Cooking Time: 8 hours

---

2 pounds (907g) Grass-Fed Lamb Roast (bone-in)

1 cup Black Olives, pitted and sliced

1 Head Garlic, peeled and smashed

½ tablespoon Dried Oregano, crushed

½ tablespoon Dried Thyme, crushed

Flaked Sea Salt, to taste

Freshly Ground Black Pepper, to taste

1 cup Homemade Low-sodium Chicken Broth

Directions:

1. Place the lamb into a slow cooker. Top the lamb with the garlic, salt, olives and black pepper.

2. Pour the broth around the lamb and sprinkle with herbs.

3. Set the slow cooker on low. Cover and cook for about 8 hours.

Nutty Ground Lamb

Ground lamb meat, almonds and spices combine to make a delicious meal. Fresh mint and cilantro adds a nice aromatic touch to the meat. Top with chopped almonds.

Servings: 4
Prep Time: 15 minutes
Cooking Time: 4 hours, 15 minutes

---

1 tablespoon Extra Virgin Coconut Oil

1 medium Onion, chopped

2 tablespoons Almonds, sliced

2 Garlic Cloves, chopped

1 Green chili, chopped

1 pound (454g) Grass-Fed Lean Ground Lamb

¼ teaspoon ground Turmeric

1 teaspoon Ground Cumin

1 teaspoon Ground Cilantro

½ teaspoon Smoked Paprika

½ teaspoon Red Pepper Flakes, crushed

Flaked Sea Salt, to taste

Freshly Ground Black Pepper, to taste

1 tablespoon diced Fresh Cilantro Leaves

2 tablespoons diced Fresh Mint Leaves

Directions:

1. In a skillet, heat the oil on a medium-high heat. Add the onion and almonds, and sauté for 4 to 5 minutes. Add the garlic and chili, and sauté for 3 to 2 minutes. Add the ground lamb and spices, and cook for 6 to 8 minutes. Transfer the lamb mixture into a slow cooker.

2. Set the slow cooker on low. Cover and cook for about 3½ hours.

3. Open the slow cooker and stir in the cilantro and mint leaves. Cook, covered, for a further 30 minutes.

4.

CASSEROLES

Cheesy Green Bean Casserole

This is a classic spin on a simple vegetable casserole. The addition of cheese and coconut milk adds a wonderful flavor to these vegetables. Top with lemon slices.

Servings: 4
Prep Time: 15 minutes
Cooking Time: 4 hours

---

1 pound (454g) Fresh Green Beans, trimmed

½ cup Mushrooms, sliced

¼ cup Onion, chopped finely

1 cup Coconut Milk

¾ cup Parmesan Cheese, shredded

Flaked Sea Salt, to taste

Freshly Ground Black Pepper, to taste

Directions:
1. In a slow cooker, mix together all of the ingredients.

2. Set the slow cooker on low. Cover and cook for 3 to 4 hours.

Florets Casserole

This is one of the simplest and easiest casserole recipes. Dried herbs and seasoning compliments the cauliflower nicely. Serve with fresh greens.

Servings: 4
Prep Time: 15 minutes
Cooking Time: 3 hours, 30 minutes

---

1 large Head Cauliflower, cut into florets

1½ cups Tomatoes, diced

1 cup Red Onion, diced

2 Garlic Cloves, minced

¾ cup Homemade Low-sodium Chicken Broth

1 teaspoon Dried Thyme, crushed

1 teaspoon Dried Oregano, crushed

¼ teaspoon Red Pepper Flakes, crushed

Flaked Sea Salt, to taste

Freshly Ground Black Pepper, to taste

Directions:

1. In a slow cooker, mix together all of the ingredients.

2. Set the slow cooker on high. Cover and cook for about 3½ hours.

Vegetable Medley Casserole

This recipe makes a satisfying and healthy, colorful vegetable casserole. The wonderful combination of vegetables and spice makes a tasty meal. Garnish with freshly chopped basil.

Servings: 4
Prep Time: 15 minutes
Cooking Time: 4 hours, 7 minutes

---

2 tablespoons Coconut Oil, Extra Virgin

1 large White Onion, chopped

2 Garlic Cloves, minced

2 large Zucchinis, diced

1 Red Bell Pepper, seeded and diced

1 Green Bell Pepper, seeded and diced

1 Orange Bell Pepper, seeded and diced

½ cup Homemade Low-sodium Vegetable Broth

2 cups Tomatoes, diced

¼ teaspoon Red Pepper Flakes, crushed

Pinch of Cayenne Pepper

Flaked Sea Salt, to taste

Freshly Ground Black Pepper, to taste

Directions:

1. In a skillet, heat the oil on a medium heat. Sauté the onion and garlic for 4 to 5 minutes. Add the bell pepper and zucchini, and sauté for a further 2 minutes.

2. Add the remaining ingredients to the skillet. Bring to the boil before transferring the vegetable mixture into a slow cooker.

3. Set the slow cooker on high. Cover and cook for 3 to 4 hours.

Mushroom Pork Casserole

This is a hearty, one-pot meal for the whole family. This casserole is easy to assemble and rich in flavors. Top with fresh cilantro leaves.

Servings: 4
Prep Time: 15 minutes
Cooking Time: 6 hours

---

4 Pork Chops, diced

2 cups Fresh Spinach, torn

2 cups Mushrooms, diced

1 White Onion, diced

2 Garlic Cloves, minced

2 cups Tomatoes, diced

2 tablespoons Homemade Tomato Paste

1 cup Homemade Low-sodium Chicken Broth

Flaked Sea Salt, to taste

Freshly Ground Black Pepper, to taste

Directions:

1. In a slow cooker, mix together all of the ingredients.

2. Set the slow cooker on high. Cover and cook for 5 to 6 hours.

Pork & Apple Pleasure

The sweetness of the apple in this recipe compliments nicely with the pork chops and other ingredients in this casserole. Enjoy with steamed vegetables.

Servings: 4
Prep Time: 15 minutes
Cooking Time: 8 hours

---

2 medium Onions, sliced

3 Apples, peeled, cored and sliced

4 Pork Chops

1 teaspoon Fresh Rosemary, chopped

1 teaspoon Dijon Mustard

2 cups Homemade Low-sodium Chicken Broth

2 tablespoons Fresh Lemon Juice

Flaked Sea Salt, to taste

Freshly Ground Black Pepper, to taste

Directions:

1. Place the onions in a slow cooker. Arrange the apple slices over the onions. Top with the chops and sprinkle with the rosemary.

2. In a bowl, mix together the mustard, broth, lemon juice, salt and black pepper. Pour the broth mixture over the

chops.

3. Set the slow cooker on low. Cover and cook for about 8 hours.

Chicken Mix Casserole

This hearty and delicious casserole is filled with the flavors of chicken, vegetables and apples. Enjoy with steamed kale.

Servings: 4
Prep Time: 15 minutes
Cooking Time: 6 hours

---

4 Grass-Fed skinless, boneless Chicken Thighs

1 large Head Broccoli, cut into florets

3 large Turnips, peeled and sliced

2 Celery Stalks, sliced

3 Apples, peeled, cored and sliced

1 Bay Leaf

1 Cinnamon Stick

Flaked Sea Salt, to taste

Freshly Ground Black Pepper, to taste

2 cups Homemade Low-sodium Chicken Broth

1½ tablespoons Arrowroot powder

3 tablespoons Water

Directions:

1. In a slow cooker, mix together all of the ingredients, except for the arrowroot and water.

2. Set the slow cooker on high. Cover and cook for 5 to 6 hours.

3. In a bowl, mix together the arrowroot and water. Stir in arrowroot mixture and switch off the slow cooker.

4. Discard the bay leaf and cinnamon stick before serving.

Chicken Squash

This tasty chicken and butternut squash casserole is filling and healthy too. The combination of ingredients works well to deliver a brain healthy dish. Serve with fresh greens.

Servings: 4
Prep Time: 15 minutes
Cooking Time: 7 hours

---

2 medium Onions, chopped finely

1 pound (454g) skinless, boneless Chicken pieces

1 pound (454g) cubed Butternut Squash

1½ cups Tomatoes, diced

1 cup Homemade Low-sodium Chicken Broth

1 tablespoon Coconut Oil, Extra Virgin

2 tablespoons Homemade Tomato Paste

1½ tablespoons Dijon Mustard

1 teaspoon Dried Thyme, crushed

1 teaspoon Dried Oregano, crushed

Flaked Sea Salt, to taste

Freshly Ground Black Pepper, to taste

1 cup Button Mushrooms, sliced

1tablespoons Arrowroot powder

2 tablespoons Water

Directions:

1. Place the onions in a slow cooker. Place the chicken, butternut squash and tomatoes over the onion. In a bowl, mix together the broth, oil, tomato paste, mustard, herbs and seasoning. Pour the broth mixture over the chicken.

2. Set the slow cooker on low. Cover and cook for 5 to 6 hours.

3. Open the slow cooker and add the mushrooms. Cover and cook for a further hour.

4. In a bowl, mix together the arrowroot and water. Stir in the arrowroot mixture and switch off the slow cooker.

Layered Cheesy Chicken

This one-dish wonder features moist, tender chicken breasts which are covered with eggplants, spinach and goat cheese. Top with freshly chopped parsley leaves.

Servings: 4
Prep Time: 20 minutes
Cooking Time: 5 hours

1½ pounds (680g) skinless, boneless Chicken Breasts, cut into chunks and pounded slightly

¾ cup Homemade Low-sodium Chicken Broth

1 medium White Onion, sliced thinly

2 Garlic Cloves, minced

¼ teaspoon Smoked Paprika

¼ teaspoon Red Pepper Flakes, crushed

Flaked Sea Salt, to taste

Freshly Ground Black Pepper, to taste

2 tablespoons Fresh Rosemary, chopped

1 medium Eggplant, sliced

3 cups Baby Spinach

1 cup Goat Cheese, crumbled

Directions:

1. In a large bowl, mix together the chicken, broth, onion, garlic, spices and rosemary.

2. In a slow cooker, add half of the chicken mixture. Place half of the eggplant slices over the chicken, and arrange on top half of the spinach leaves. Top with half of the cheese. Repeat the layer.

3. Set the slow cooker on low. Cover and cook for about 5 hours.

Pumpkin Beef Casserole

This dish makes one of the best comfort meals for the whole family. This dish is a perfect family meal for a chilly day. Serve with fresh greens.

Servings: 4
Prep Time: 20 minutes
Cooking Time: 6 hours, 41 minutes

---

1 tablespoon Extra Virgin Olive Oil

1 pound (454g) Grass-Fed Lean Ground Beef

1 White Onion, chopped

2 Garlic Cloves, minced

1 cup Celery Stalk, chopped

1 cup Green Beans, trimmed and halved

1 tablespoon Fresh Thyme, chopped

1 tablespoon Fresh Oregano, chopped

¼ teaspoon Smoked Paprika

¼ teaspoon Red Pepper Flakes, crushed

Flaked Sea Salt, to taste

Freshly Ground Black Pepper, to taste

½ cup Homemade Low-sodium Beef Broth

3 cups Cooked Pumpkin, mashed

Directions:

1. In a skillet, heat the oil on a medium heat. Add the beef and cook for 4 to 5 minutes. Transfer the beef into a slow cooker.

2. In the same skillet, add the onion, garlic, celery and sauté for 4 to 5 minutes. Add the beans, herbs and spices, and sauté for a further minute. Transfer the onion mixture into the slow cooker and mix with the beef.

3. Add the broth and top with mashed pumpkin. Set the slow cooker on low. Cover and cook for 5 to 6 hours.

4. Uncover the slow cooker and turn to high. Cook for a further 30 minutes.

Winter Beef Casserole

The squash used in this recipe combines nicely with the beef. This casserole is also a great way to use up the bounty of squash in the garden. Top with freshly chopped basil leaves.

Servings: 4
Prep Time: 20 minutes
Cooking Time: 5 hours, 10 minutes

---

1 tablespoon Extra Virgin Olive Oil

2 Yellow Onions, chopped

3 Celery Stalks, diced

4 Garlic Cloves, minced

1 pound (454g) Grass-Fed Beef Chunks

4 Winter Squash, cubed

2 cups Tomatoes, diced

2 tablespoons Homemade Tomato Puree

2 Bay Leaves

1 tablespoon Fresh Lemon Juice

2 cups Homemade Low-sodium Beef Broth

Directions:

1. In a skillet, heat the oil on a medium heat. Add the onion, celery and garlic, and sauté for 4 to 5 minutes. Add the beef and cook for 4 to 5 minutes. Transfer the beef

mixture into a slow cooker.

2. Add the remaining ingredients and mix well.

3. Set the slow cooker on high. Cover and cook for 4 to 5 hours.

SOUP RECIPES

Spetetti Beef Cabbage Soup

This is a spectacular and delicious beef soup for a soup day. This hearty soup could quickly become a crowd pleaser. Garnish with chopped fresh scallion leaves.

Servings: 4
Prep Time: 20 minutes
Cooking Time: 8 hours

---

1 teaspoon Extra Virgin Olive Oil

½ pound (226g) Grass-Fed Lean Ground Beef

1 small White Onion, chopped

1 Garlic Clove, minced

3 cups Cabbage, chopped

1 Bay Leaf

⅛ teaspoon Celery Seeds

¼ teaspoon Smoked Paprika

¼ teaspoon Red Pepper Flakes, crushed

½ teaspoon Ground Cumin

2 cups Homemade Low-sodium Beef Broth

Flaked Sea Salt, to taste

Freshly Ground Black Pepper, to taste

Directions:

1. In a skillet, heat the oil on a medium heat. Add the beef and cook for 4 to 5 minutes. Drain the beef and transfer onto a plate. In the same skillet, add the onion, garlic, cabbage, bay leaf, celery seeds and spices and sauté for about 2 minutes.

2. Transfer the beef and cabbage mixture into a slow cooker. Pour over the broth and season with salt and black pepper.

3. Set the slow cooker on low. Cover and cook for 8 hours.

Beef & Mushrooms Soup

This warming beef and mushroom soup is great as a starter for a lavish dinner and may quickly become a family favorite. Serve with a drizzling of fresh lemon juice.

Servings: 4
Prep Time: 15 minutes
Cooking Time: 6-8 hours, 5 minutes

---

1 pound (454g) Grass-Fed Beef Stew Meat

½ teaspoon Chili Powder

2 tablespoon Arrowroot Starch

1 tablespoon Extra Virgin Olive Oil

1 small White Onion, chopped

1 Celery Stalk, chopped

1 teaspoon Dried Thyme, crushed

2 cups White Mushrooms, chopped

2½ cups Homemade Low-sodium Beef Broth

Flaked Sea Salt, to taste

Freshly Ground Black Pepper, to taste

Directions:

1. In a bowl, mix together the beef, chili powder and arrowroot starch. In a skillet, heat the oil on a high heat. Add the beef, onion and celery and cook for 4 to 5 minutes. Remove from the heat and stir in the thyme.

2. Place the mushrooms into a slow cooker, and place the beef mixture over the mushrooms. Pour in the broth and season with salt and black pepper.

3. Set the slow cooker on low. Cover and cook for 6-8 hours.

Healthy Chicken Soup

This easy recipe makes a healthy yet delicious soup which will be soothing your stomach. Serve with grated parmesan cheese sprinkled on top.

Servings: 4
Prep Time: 10 minutes
Cooking Time: 8 hours, 30 minutes

---

4 Grass-Fed skinless Chicken Legs

2 medium Butternut Squash, sliced

2 medium Zucchini, sliced

1 cup Fresh Green Beans, trimmed and chopped

2 Celery Stalks, chopped

1 small Yellow Onion, chopped

1 Garlic Clove, chopped

1 Bay Leaf

2 Sprigs Fresh Oregano

1 tablespoon Fresh Lime Juice

3 cups Homemade Low-sodium Chicken Broth

1 teaspoon Dried Basil, crushed

Flaked Sea Salt, to taste

Freshly Ground Black Pepper, to taste

Directions:

1. Mix together all of the ingredients in a slow cooker.

2. Set the slow cooker on low. Cover and cook for 8 hours.

3. Remove the chicken legs and oregano sprigs. Remove the meat from the bones and shred it before returning the meat to the soup.

4. Cover and cook for a further 30 minutes.

Belled Chicken Soup

This chicken and bell pepper soup is not only mouthwatering, it is also quite healthy and easy to prepare. Garnish with freshly chopped parsley leaves.

Servings: 4
Prep Time: 15 minutes
Cooking Time: 5 hours, 15 minutes

½ tablespoon Extra Virgin Olive Oil

1 small White Onion, chopped

2 Celery Stalks, chopped

1 Green Bell pepper, seeded and chopped

1 Red Bell Pepper, seeded and chopped

1 tablespoon Garlic, diced

2 cups cooked Grass-Fed Chicken, shredded

2 cups Homemade Low-sodium Chicken Broth

2 tablespoons Fresh Parsley, chopped

2 tablespoons Scallions, chopped

Flaked Sea Salt, to taste

Freshly Ground Black Pepper, to taste

Directions:

1. In a skillet, heat the oil on a medium heat. Add the onion, celery and bell pepper and sauté for about 10 minutes. Add the garlic and sauté for 5 minutes more.

2. Transfer the onion mixture into a slow cooker. Add the remaining ingredients and mix.

3. Set the slow cooker on low. Cover and cook for 4 to 5 hours.

Chicken Burro Soup

This classic chicken soup is full of great flavors and is a perfect comfort soup. Serve with a garnishing of avocado slices.

Servings: 4
Prep Time: 15 minutes
Cooking Time: 8 hours

---

2 cups cooked Grass-Fed Chicken, shredded

½ cup Button Mushrooms, chopped

1 medium Tomato, chopped

1 small White Onion, chopped

3 tablespoons Green Chilies, diced

2 Garlic Cloves, minced

2 cups Homemade Low-sodium Chicken Broth

3 tablespoons Fresh Lime Juice

½ teaspoon Dried Thyme, crushed

¼ teaspoon Ground Cumin

Flaked Sea Salt, to taste

Freshly Ground Black Pepper, to taste

Directions:

1. Mix together all of the ingredients in a slow cooker.

2. Set the slow cooker on low. Cover and cook for 8 hours.

Herbed Chicken Soup

This soup is chock full of chicken and wonderful herb flavors. It would make a great evening meal for the whole family. Top with freshly grated lemon zest.

Servings: 4
Prep Time: 15 minutes
Cooking Time: 8 hours

---

1 small White Onion, chopped

2 large Zucchini, chopped

3 Celery Stalks, chopped

1 teaspoon Fresh Lemon Juice

2 Fresh Thyme Sprigs

2 Fresh Oregano Sprigs

2 Grass-Fed boneless, diced, Chicken Thighs

2½ cups Homemade Low-sodium Chicken Broth

Flaked Sea Salt, to taste

Freshly Ground Black Pepper, to taste

Directions:

1. Mix together all of the ingredients in a slow cooker.

2. Set the slow cooker on low. Cover and cook for 8 hours.

3. Discard the herb sprigs before serving.

Chicken & Spinach Combo

This delicious soup is great for your body and soul. The lemon used in this recipe really brightens this soup's flavor nicely. Top with freshly chopped basil leaves.

Servings: 4
Prep Time: 15 minutes
Cooking Time: 6 hours

---

3 cups Homemade Low-sodium Chicken Broth

¼ cup Extra Virgin Olive Oil

½ cup White Onion, chopped

2 cups cooked Grass-Fed Chicken, shredded

1 Bunch Fresh Spinach, chopped

2 teaspoons Lemon Zest, grated freshly

1½ tablespoons Fresh Lemon Juice

Flaked Sea Salt, to taste

Freshly Ground Black Pepper, to taste

Directions:

1. In a blender, add 1 cup of the broth, the oil and onion and pulse until smooth. Transfer the mixture into a slow

cooker. Add the remaining ingredients and mix.

2. Set the slow cooker on low. Cover and cook for 6 hours.

Creamy Chicken Soup

This recipe not only makes an easy and delicious soup, the spices and coconut milk also provides a unique taste. Serve with a drizzle of fresh lime juice.

Servings: 4
Prep Time: 15 minutes
Cooking Time: 5 hours

---

1 pound (454g) Grass-Fed boneless, diced, Chicken Thighs1 Head Cabbage, chopped

1 medium Onion, chopped

1 Garlic Clove, minced

½ cup Green Chilies, chopped

2 cups Homemade Low-sodium Chicken Broth

¼ teaspoon Ground Cilantro

½ teaspoon Ground Cumin

Flaked Sea Salt, to taste

Freshly Ground Black Pepper, to taste

1½ tablespoons Coconut Flour

½ cup fresh Coconut Milk, unsweetened

Directions:

1. In a slow cooker, mix together all of the ingredients, except for the coconut flour and milk.

2. Set the slow cooker on low. Cover and cook for 5 hours.

3. In the last 10 minutes add the coconut flour and milk whilst continuously stirring.

Green Chicken Soup

This chicken soup is loaded with healthy nutrients, and is perfect for easy weeknight dinners during the winter and the flu season. Top with freshly chopped scallion.

Servings: 4
Prep Time: 15 minutes
Cooking Time: 7 hours

---

1 pound (454g) Grass-Fed boneless, diced, Chicken Breast

1 medium Onion, chopped

2 Celery Stalks, chopped

1 Garlic Clove, minced

2 cups Homemade Low-sodium Chicken Broth

4 cups Fresh Collard Greens, chopped

1 teaspoon Dried Oregano, crushed

Flaked Sea Salt, to taste

Freshly Ground Black Pepper, to taste

Directions:

1. In a slow cooker, add the chicken, celery, onion, garlic and broth.

2. Set the slow cooker on low. Cover and cook for 5 to 6 hours.

3. Add the remaining ingredients and cook for a further hour.

Spicy Jambalaya Soup

This rich spicy soup is hearty and filling. It has a twist of flavors from the different peppers and other spices. Serve with a sprinkle of fresh lemon juice.

Servings: 4
Prep Time: 15 minutes
Cooking Time: 6 hours

½ pound (226g) Grass-Fed boneless, diced Chicken

1 Green Bell Pepper, seeded and chopped

1 Yellow Bell Pepper, seeded and chopped

1 cup Tomatoes, chopped

1 medium Onion, chopped

1 Garlic Clove, minced

1 Bay Leaf

¼ teaspoon Smoked Paprika

¼ teaspoon Cayenne Pepper

¼ teaspoon Red Pepper Flakes, crushed

Flaked Sea Salt, to taste

Freshly Ground Black Pepper, to taste

3 cups Homemade Low-sodium Chicken Broth

½ pound (226g) Raw Shrimp, peeled and deveined

½ Head Cauliflower, chopped like rice consistency

Directions:

1. In a slow cooker, mix together all of the ingredients, except for the Shrimp and cauliflower.

2. Set the slow cooker on low. Cover and cook for 6 hours.

3. In the last 20 minutes stir in shrimp and cauliflower rice.

Salmon Reef Soup

This dish combines the wonderful tastes of salmon and turnip. This soup is filling and packed with lots of nutrients. Drizzle with fresh lemon juice before serving.

Servings: 4
Prep Time: 15 minutes
Cooking Time: 10 hours 15 minutes

---

1 pound (454g) Salmon Fillets

2 medium Yellow Squash, chopped

2 Celery Stalks, chopped

6 Turnips, peeled and chopped

1 small White Onion, chopped

½ tablespoon Garlic, minced

1 teaspoon Red Pepper Flakes, crushed

2 cups Homemade Low-sodium Chicken Broth

1 cup Coconut Milk, unsweetened

Flaked Sea Salt, to taste

Freshly Ground Black Pepper, to taste

Directions:

1. In a slow cooker, mix together the fish, vegetables, red pepper flakes and broth.

2. Set the slow cooker on low. Cover and cook for 10 hours.

3. Once cooked, cool the soup slightly. Transfer the soup into a blender and pulse until smooth.

4. Return the soup into a large pan. Add the coconut milk and cook for a further 4 to 5 minutes. Season with salt and black pepper before serving.

Seafood Mania Soup

This authentic soup is incredible in flavor. The combination of spices and coconut milk adds a wonderful flavoring to the fish and shrimp. Top with freshly grated lemon zest.

Servings: 4
Prep Time: 15 minutes
Cooking Time: 8 hours, 20 minutes

½ pound (226g) Cod Fillets

1 tablespoon Extra Virgin Olive Oil

1 Scallion, chopped

1 medium Onion, chopped

2 Celery Stalks, chopped

1 large Head of Cabbage, chopped

¼ teaspoon Dried Oregano, crushed

1 Bay Leaf

¼ teaspoon Cayenne Pepper

¼ teaspoon Red Pepper Flakes, crushed

Flaked Sea Salt, to taste

Freshly Ground Black Pepper, to taste

3 cups Homemade Low-sodium Chicken Broth

½ pound (226g) Raw Shrimp, peeled and deveined

½ cup Coconut Milk, unsweetened

Directions:

1. In a skillet, heat the oil on a medium heat. Add the scallion, onion and celery and sauté for about 10 minutes. Transfer the mixture into a slow cooker. Mix the remaining ingredients, except for the shrimp, into the slow cooker.

2. Set the slow cooker on low. Cover and cook for 6 - 8 hours.

3. Once cooked, stir in shrimp and coconut milk. Set the slow cooker on high. Cover and cook for a further 10 minutes.

Mushroom Grandeur Soup

This tasty soup is filled with the hearty flavors and nutrients of mushrooms. Enjoy the fabulous flavor while you boost your whole family is sure to love. Garnish with freshly chopped parsley.

Servings: 4
Prep Time: 15 minutes
Cooking Time: 4 hours 11 minutes

---

1 teaspoon Extra Virgin Olive Oil

1 small White Onion, chopped

1 Garlic Clove, minced

½ cup Portobello Mushrooms, sliced

½ cup Button Mushrooms, sliced

1 Bay Leaf

½ teaspoon Fresh Oregano, chopped

½ teaspoon Fresh Thyme, chopped

1½ cups Homemade Low-sodium Beef Broth

Flaked Sea Salt, to taste

Freshly Ground Black Pepper, to taste

½ teaspoon Arrowroot Powder

½ cup Coconut Milk, unsweetened

Directions:

1. In a skillet, heat the oil on a medium heat. Add the garlic, onion and mushrooms, and sauté for 4 to 5 minutes. Stir in the bay leaf, oregano and thyme and cook for 1 minute more.

2. Transfer the mixture into a slow cooker. Pour in the broth and season with salt and black pepper. Set the slow cooker on low. Cover and cook for 4 hours.

3. In a bowl, mix together the arrowroot and coconut milk. Uncover the slow cooker and add the milk mixture to the soup, stirring continuously. For the final 5 minutes cook the soup whilst stirring occasionally.

Tomato Glee Soup

This wonderful soup is a great classic for your slow cooker. The chicken broth and fresh herbs nicely goes with the tomatoes. Garnish with chopped scallion.

Servings: 4
Prep Time: 15 minutes
Cooking Time: 4 hours

---

2 cups Tomatoes, chopped

½ cup Homemade Tomato Paste

1 cup Fresh Kale, trimmed and chopped

1 small Yellow Onion, chopped

1 Garlic Clove, minced

½ tablespoon Fresh Thyme, chopped

½ tablespoon Fresh Oregano, chopped

2 cups Homemade Low-sodium Chicken Broth

Flaked Sea Salt, to taste

Freshly Ground Black Pepper, to taste

Directions:

1. Mix together all of the ingredients in a slow cooker.

2. Set the slow cooker on low. Cover and cook for 4 hours.

Coconut Onion Soup

This is a healthy and authentic soup which is full of wonderful flavors of the coconut oil and onion. Serve with a sprinkling of crushed red pepper flakes.

Servings: 4
Prep Time: 10 minutes
Cooking Time: 22 hours

1 pound (454g) Sweet Onion, sliced thinly

1 tablespoon Extra Virgin Coconut Oil

1 teaspoon Dried Oregano, crushed

1½ cups Homemade Low-sodium Chicken Broth

1½ cups Homemade Low-sodium Beef Broth

Flaked Sea Salt, to taste

Freshly Ground Black Pepper, to taste

Directions:

1. Add the onion and oil to a slow cooker. Set the slow cooker on high for caramelizing. Cover and cook for 10 to 12 hours.

2. Open the slow cooker and add the remaining ingredients

before setting the temperature to low.

3. Cover and cook for a further 8 to 10 hours.

Spiced Pumpkin Soup

This hearty vegetable soup will warm you up whenever you need it most. The spices used in this dish have added a nice spark to the soup. Top with freshly chopped scallion.

Servings: 4
Prep Time: 15 minutes
Cooking Time: 8 hours

---

1 tablespoon Extra Virgin Olive Oil

1 medium Onion, chopped

½ tablespoon Fresh Ginger, minced

1 Garlic Clove, minced

½ teaspoon Ground Cilantro

½ teaspoon Ground Cumin

¼ teaspoon Red Pepper Flakes, crushed

1 medium Pumpkin, peeled, seeded and chopped

3 Turnips, peeled and chopped

3 cups Homemade Low-sodium Vegetable Broth

Flaked Sea Salt, to taste

Freshly Ground Black Pepper, to taste

Directions:

1. In a skillet, heat the oil on a medium heat. Add the onion, ginger and garlic and sauté for 6 to 8 minutes. Add the spices and sauté for 2 minutes more. Transfer the mixture into a slow cooker.

2. Add the remaining ingredients to the slow cooker and mix together.

3. Set the slow cooker on low. Cover and cook for 6 to 8 hours.

STEW RECIPES

Pepron Beef Veggie Stew

This stew nicely combines hearty beef with vegetables and broth. This delicious stew will warm you up on a cold winter evening or whenever you wish. Top the completed dish with grated parmesan cheese.

Servings: 4
Prep Time: 20 minutes
Cooking Time: 8 hours, 5 minutes

---

1 tablespoon Extra Virgin Olive Oil

1 pound (454g) Grass-Fed Stewing Beef

½ cup Fresh Mushrooms, quartered

¼ cup Green Bell Pepper, seeded and chopped

2 Celery Ribs, chopped

1 cup Tomatoes, chopped

1 small White Onion, chopped

2 Garlic Cloves, minced

2 tablespoons Homemade Tomato Paste

1¼ cups Homemade Low-sodium Beef Broth

1 teaspoon Dried Thyme, crushed

Flaked Sea Salt, to taste

Freshly Ground Black Pepper, to taste

Directions:

1. In a skillet, heat the oil on a medium heat. Add the beef and cook for 4 to 5 minutes.

2. Mix together the beef and the remaining ingredients in a slow cooker.

3. Set the slow cooker on low. Cover and cook for 6 to 8 hours.

Swiss Beef Stew

This beef and Swiss chard combines beautifully to make a luxurious and brain healthy dish for a family dinner. Top it with freshly grated lime zest.

Servings: 4
Prep Time: 20 minutes (plus time to marinate)
Cooking Time: 12 hours, 16 minutes

---

1 pound (454g) Grass-Fed Stewing Beef, diced into 1-inch pieces

¼ cup Extra Virgin Olive Oil

3 Garlic Cloves, minced

1 medium White Onion, chopped

1 Jalapeño Pepper, seeded and chopped

1½ cups Homemade Low-sodium Beef Broth

1 large bunch Swiss Chard, trimmed and chopped

Flaked Sea Salt, to taste

Freshly Ground Black Pepper, to taste

Directions:

1. In a bowl, add the beef and garlic, and coat with 2 tablespoon of the oil. Cover and refrigerate for 6 to 8

hours. In a skillet, heat 1 tablespoon of oil on a medium heat. Add the beef and cook for 4 to 5 minutes. Transfer the beef onto a plate

2. In the same skillet, heat the remaining oil on a medium heat. Add the onion and sauté for about 10 minutes. Add the jalapeño and sauté for 1 minute more.

3. Transfer the beef, onion mixture and broth into a slow cooker and mix. Set the slow cooker on low. Cover and cook for 10 hours.

4. Open the slow cooker and stir in the Swiss chard, salt and black pepper. Cover and cook for 2 hours more.

Chili Beef Stew

*This is a hearty and delicious beef stew. The combination of
vegetables and spices makes this a wonderfully flavored spicy dish.
Serve with a drizzle of fresh lemon juice.*

Servings: 4
Prep Time: 20 minutes
Cooking Time: 8 hours, 15 minutes

---

2 tablespoons Extra Virgin Olive Oil

½ pound (226g) Grass-Fed Ground Beef

½ pound (226g) Grass-Fed Stewing Beef

1½ tablespoons Chili Powder

3 Garlic Cloves, minced

1 small White Onion, chopped

1 small Yellow Squash, chopped

1 cup Fresh Mushrooms, sliced

½ tablespoon Ground Cilantro

½ tablespoon Ground Cumin

Flaked Sea Salt, to taste

Freshly Ground Black Pepper, to taste

1½ cups Homemade Tomato Paste

1½ cups Homemade Low-sodium Beef Broth

Directions:

1. In a skillet, heat ½ tablespoon of oil on a medium-high heat. Add the ground beef and cook for 4 to 5 minutes. Transfer the ground beef into a slow cooker. In the same skillet, heat another ½ tablespoon of oil on a medium-high heat. Add the stewing beef and ½ tablespoon of chili powder, and sauté for 4 to 5 minutes. Transfer the beef into the slow cooker.

2. Heat the remaining oil on a medium heat. Add the garlic, onion, squash and mushrooms, and sauté for 4 to 5 minutes. Transfer the vegetable mixture into the slow cooker.

3. In the slow cooker, mix in the spices, tomato paste and broth.

4. Set the slow cooker on low. Cover and cook for 8 hours.

Garlic Shank Stew

The delicately flavored broth used in this recipe combines wonderfully with the beef shanks and cabbage to create a delicious dish, ideal for an interestingly healthy dinner. Garnish with fresh cilantro leaves.

Servings: 4
Prep Time: 20 minutes
Cooking Time: 9 hours

---

2 small Onions, sliced

2 Celery Stalks, chopped

1 small Head Cabbage, cored and cut into 8 wedges

1 Bay Leaf

6 Garlic Cloves, minced

2 (2-inch thick) Grass-Fed Beef Shanks

Flaked Sea Salt, to taste

Freshly Ground Black Pepper, to taste

½ teaspoon Red Pepper Flakes, crushed

1½ cups Tomatoes, diced

1 cup Homemade Low-sodium Beef Broth

Directions:

1. In a slow cooker, place the onion, celery, cabbage, bay leaf and garlic.

2. Generously sprinkle the beef shanks with salt and black pepper. Place the shanks on top of the vegetables and add the remaining ingredients.

3. Set the slow cooker on low. Cover and cook for 9 hours.

Herbed Lamb Stew

This delicious and aromatic stew is full of fresh flavors. It is ideal for sharing with your family or guests. Garnish with avocado slices.

Servings: 4
Prep Time: 20 minutes
Cooking Time: 6 hours

---

1 pound (454g) Grass-Fed Lamb Stewing Meat

¼ cup Extra Virgin Olive Oil

2 Garlic Cloves, minced

1 medium White Onion, chopped

3 large Turnips, peeled and diced

3 Celery Stalks, diced

2 cups Fresh Green Beans

1 Bay Leaf

2 Fresh Thyme Sprigs

1 tablespoon Fresh Cilantro, chopped

1 teaspoon Fresh Lemon Juice

1½ cups Water

Flaked Sea Salt, to taste

Freshly Ground Black Pepper, to taste

Directions:

1. In a slow cooker, mix together all of the ingredients.

2. Set the slow cooker on low. Cover and cook for 6 hours.

3. Remove the thyme sprigs before serving.

Spicy Lamb Stew

Warm spices and dried herbs compliment the lamb and mushroom in this recipe very well. You will also enjoy the amazing smell of this dish which will fill your house. Top with freshly chopped cilantro.

Servings: 4
Prep Time: 20 minutes
Cooking Time: 10 hours

1½ cups Homemade Low-sodium Chicken Broth

1 cup Tomatoes, diced

2 Green Chilies, seeded and sliced

1½ pounds (680g) Grass-Fed Lamb Shoulders and Neck Bones

3 Garlic Cloves, minced

1 small White Onion, chopped

1 tablespoon Fresh Lemon Juice

½ teaspoon Ground Cumin

¼ teaspoon Ground Cinnamon

½ tablespoon Dried Thyme, crushed

½ tablespoon Dried Oregano, crushed

Flaked Sea Salt, to taste

Freshly Ground Black Pepper, to taste

1 cup Fresh White Mushrooms, sliced

Directions:

1. In a blender, add ½ cup of broth, tomatoes and chilies, and pulse until smooth. Transfer the tomato mixture into a slow cooker.

2. Add the remaining broth and, apart for the mushrooms, the remaining ingredients.

3. Set the slow cooker on low. Cover and cook for 8 hours.

4. Open the slow cooker and stir in mushrooms. Cover and cook for a further 2 hours.

Chicken & Zucchini Stew

This spicy chicken stew uses simple ingredients to make a hearty and filling meal. The spices used in this recipe helps to create a wonderful aroma during the cooking process. Garnish with freshly grated lemon zest.

Servings: 4
Prep Time: 15 minutes
Cooking Time: 4 hours

---

1 pound (454g) Grass-Fed boneless Chicken Thighs

1 small Onion, chopped

2 Garlic Cloves, minced

2 Celery Stalks, diced

2 Zucchinis, diced

1½ cups Tomatoes, diced

1 teaspoon Fresh Lemon juice

1 teaspoon Ground Cumin

½ teaspoon Ground Cilantro

½ tablespoon Ground Turmeric

½ tablespoon Dried Thyme, crushed

Flaked Sea Salt, to taste

Freshly Ground Black Pepper, to taste

1¼ cups Homemade Low-sodium Chicken Broth

Directions:

1. Mix together all of the ingredients in the slow cooker.

2. Set the slow cooker on high. Cover and cook for 4 hours.

Chicken Verde Stew

This is one of the best stress-free recipes which work well if you are catering for guests. The spinach adds a beautiful color and many essential nutrients to this chicken stew. Serve with shredded parmesan cheese.

Servings: 4
Prep Time: 15 minutes
Cooking Time: 8 hours

---

1 pound (454g) Grass-Fed boneless Chicken Breasts

1 medium Onion, chopped

2 Celery Stalks, chopped

Flaked Sea Salt, to taste

Freshly Ground Black Pepper, to taste

1 tablespoon Homemade Tomato Paste

1¼ cups Homemade Low-sodium Chicken Broth

4 cups Fresh Spinach, chopped

Directions:

1. Mix together all of the ingredients, except the spinach, in a slow cooker.

2. Set the slow cooker on low. Cover and cook for 6 to 7 hours.

3. Open the slow cooker and stir in spinach. Cover and cook for 1 hour more.

Hearty Chicken Stew

This recipe makes a great tasting meal that your whole family will love. Chicken and vegetables combine to make a tasty, hearty stew. Garnish with lemon slices.

Servings: 4
Prep Time: 15 minutes
Cooking Time: 5 hours

---

1 pound (454g) diced Grass-Fed boneless Chicken Breasts

2 cups Cabbage, chopped

1 medium Onion, chopped

3 Celery Stalks, chopped

2 cups Tomatoes, diced

1 cup Homemade Low-sodium Chicken Broth

Flaked Sea Salt, to taste

Freshly Ground Black Pepper, to taste

3 cups Fresh Kale, trimmed and chopped

Directions:

1. In a slow cooker, apart for the kale, mix together all of the ingredients.

2. Set the slow cooker on high. Cover and cook for 3½ hours.

3. Open the slow cooker and stir in the kale. Cover and cook for a further 1½ hours.

Turkey Tomato Stew

This hearty and tasty stew is filled with the flavors of turkey, tomatoes and dried herbs. Garnish with freshly chopped parsley.

Servings: 4
Prep Time: 15 minutes
Cooking Time: 10 hours

1½ pounds (680g) diced Grass-Fed boneless Turkey Thigh Meat

1½ cups Tomatoes, chopped finely

1 medium Onion, sliced

¼ teaspoon Dried Oregano, crushed

¼ teaspoon Dried Thyme, crushed

Flaked Sea Salt, to taste

Freshly Ground Black Pepper, to taste

1 teaspoon Fresh Lemon Juice

1 cup Homemade Low-sodium Chicken Broth

Directions:

1. In a slow cooker, mix together all of the ingredients.

2. Set the slow cooker on low. Cover and cook for 8 to 10

hours.

Turkey Twist Stew

This is one of the simplest yet truly fabulous ground turkey stew recipes. This dish uses spices to give a wonderfully balanced flavor to the turkey and vegetables. Garnish this dish with fresh parsley.

Servings: 4
Prep Time: 15 minutes
Cooking Time: 10 hours 5 minutes

---

1 teaspoon Extra Virgin Olive Oil

1 pound (454g) Grass-Fed Lean Ground Turkey

½ cup White Onion, chopped

½ cup Celery Stalk, chopped

2 cups Fresh Mushrooms, chopped

2 cups Zucchini, chopped

1½ cup Tomatoes, diced

1 Bay Leaf

¼ teaspoon Red Pepper Flakes, crushed

¼ teaspoon Cayenne Pepper

½ teaspoon Ground Cumin

Flaked Sea Salt, to taste

Freshly Ground Black Pepper, to taste

1 cup Homemade Low-sodium Chicken Broth

Directions:

1. In a skillet, heat the oil on a medium-high heat. Add the ground turkey and cook for 4 to 5 minutes. Drain the fat and transfer the ground turkey into a slow cooker.

2. Mix the remaining ingredients into the slow cooker.

3. Set the slow cooker on low. Cover and cook for 8 to 10 hours.

Double-V Stew

This is a classic and tasty recipe which uses venison to make a comforting and filling dinner. This stew may also be a hit for winter nights. Serve with a drizzling of fresh lemon juice.

Servings: 4
Prep Time: 15 minutes
Cooking Time: 3 hours

---

1 tablespoon Extra Virgin Olive Oil

1 pound (454g) Venison Stewing Meat

2 Garlic Cloves, minced

1 medium White Onion, chopped

1½ cups Cauliflower, diced

1 cup Celery Stalk, diced

1 Bay Leaf

½ tablespoon Dried Thyme, crushed

½ tablespoon Dried Oregano, crushed

½ teaspoon Cayenne Pepper

Flaked Sea Salt, to taste

Freshly Ground Black Pepper, to taste

2 cups Low-sodium Homemade Vegetable Broth

1½ tablespoons Arrowroot Starch mixed with ½ cup water

Directions:

1. In a skillet, heat the oil on a medium-high heat. Add the venison and cook for 4 to 5 minutes.

2. Mix together the venison and the remaining ingredients in a slow cooker.

3. Set the slow cooker on high. Cover and cook for 2 to 3 hours.

DESSERTS

Cottle Pumpkin Pudding

This is a wonderfully delicious yet healthy desert for the whole family. Serve with a topping of additional nuts and unsweetened shredded coconut.

Servings: 4
Prep Time: 15 minutes
Cooking Time: 8 hours

---

3 cups Homemade Pumpkin Puree

3 Organic Eggs

3 tablespoons Coconut Flour

1 teaspoon non-aluminum, gluten free Baking Powder

2 tablespoons Coconut Oil, Extra Virgin

2 cups Coconut Milk, unsweetened

Natural Stevia, to taste

2 teaspoons Pumpkin Pie Spice

1½ teaspoons Organic Vanilla Extract

Directions:

1. Grease a slow cooker. Melt the coconut oil.

2. Mix together all of the ingredients into the prepared cooker.

3. Set the slow cooker on low. Cover and cook for 6 to 8 hours.

Chocolaty Fudge

This classic and truly yummy fudge recipe will be a special and favorite treat for lovers of chocolate. Garnish this fudge with unsweetened shredded coconut.

Servings: 4
Prep Time: 15 minutes (plus time to sit and refrigerate overnight)
Cooking Time: 2 hours

2½ cups 70% Semi Sweet Chocolate Chips

Natural Stevia, to taste

½ cup Coconut Milk, unsweetened

Pinch of Flaked Sea Salt

1 teaspoon Organic Vanilla Extract

Directions:

1. Grease a slow cooker. Except for the vanilla, mix together all of the ingredients in the cooker.

2. Set the slow cooker on high. Cover and cook for 2 hours.

3. Remove from the heat and uncover the slow cooker. Stir in the vanilla. Set aside the cooker, uncovered, for 3 to 4

hours. Stir the fudge for about 8 to 10 minutes and transfer onto a greased baking dish.

4. Refrigerate overnight. With a sharp knife, cut the fudge into bite sized pieces before serving.

Mixed Berry Cobbler

This delicious recipe is one of the best ways to use seasonal fresh berries. Serve with a topping of chopped nuts.

Servings: 4
Prep Time: 20 minutes
Cooking Time: 2 hours

½ cup Almond Flour

2 tablespoons Coconut Flour

½ teaspoon non-aluminum, gluten free Baking Soda

¼ teaspoon Ground Cinnamon

Pinch of Flaked Sea Salt

1 Organic Egg

2 tablespoons Natural Stevia

1 tablespoon Extra Virgin Coconut Oil

2 tablespoons unsweetened Almond Milk

1 cup Fresh Blackberries

1 cup Fresh Raspberries

Directions:

1. In a bowl, mix together the flours, baking soda, cinnamon and salt. In another bowl, add the eggs, stevia, oil (melted) and milk, and beat until combined. Mix the egg mixture into the flour mixture.

2. Transfer the mixture into a greased slow cooker. Evenly top with the berries.

3. Set the slow cooker on high. Cover and cook for 2 hours.

Coconut Stuffed Apples

This is a great fruity dessert for family and friend's gatherings.
Serve with a dusting of ground cinnamon.

Servings: 4
Prep Time: 15 minutes
Cooking Time: 3 hours

¼ cup unsweetened Almond Butter

¼ cup unsweetened, melted, Coconut Butter,

3 tablespoons shredded Coconut (unsweetened)

2 tablespoons Ground Cinnamon

Pinch of Flaked Sea Salt

4 Green Apples, cored (do not remove the bottom)

1 cup Water

Directions:

1. In a bowl, mix together the butters, cinnamon, coconut and salt.

2. Stuff each apple with the coconut mixture.

3. Arrange the apples in a slow cooker and pour the water around the apples.

4. Set the slow cooker on low. Cover and cook for 2 to 3 hours.

Nutty Bananas

This recipe makes one of the best and a truly delicious kid's dessert. Top these delicious bananas with whipped coconut cream.

Pear Servings: 4
Prep Time: 20 minutes
Cooking Time: 2 hours

---

8 Bananas, peeled and quartered

1 cup unsweetened Coconut Flakes

½ cup Pecans, chopped

⅓ cup Extra Virgin Coconut Oil

2 tablespoons Natural Stevia

1 teaspoon Organic Vanilla Extract

2 tablespoons Fresh Lemon juice

1 teaspoon Lemon Zest, grated freshly

½ teaspoon Ground Cinnamon

Directions:

1. Arrange the bananas in a slow cooker. Place the pecans and coconut flakes over the bananas.

2. Melt the coconut oil and mix this together with the remaining ingredients. Pour the oil mixture evenly over the bananas.

3. Set the slow cooker on low. Cover and cook for 1½ to 2 hours.

Chocolaty Mug Brownies

These brownies are simple to make and are a perfect treat for a chocolate lover. Top with chopped nuts.

Servings: 4
Prep Time: 15 minutes
Cooking Time: 1¾ hours

---

1 cup Almond Butter

2 Organic Eggs

¼ cup Organic Cocoa Powder

½ teaspoon non-aluminum, gluten free Baking Soda

¼ teaspoon Ground Cinnamon

Pinch of Flaked Sea Salt

Pinch of Ground Allspice

1 teaspoon Organic Vanilla Extract

Directions:

1. Grease a slow cooker.

2. Mix together all of the ingredients in a large bowl.

3. Transfer the mixture into 4 heatproof mugs.

4. Set the slow cooker on high. Cover and cook for 1 to 1¾ hours.

Nutty Zucchini Bread

This moist and delicious bread is packed with the flavors of zucchini, walnuts and spices. Serve with almond butter.

Servings: 4
Prep Time: 15 minutes
Cooking Time: 4 hours

---

2 cups Almond Flour

½ teaspoon non-aluminum, gluten free Baking Powder

¼ teaspoon Ground Nutmeg

1 teaspoon Ground Cinnamon

Pinch of Ground Cloves

¼ teaspoon Flaked Sea Salt

⅔ cup melted Extra Virgin Coconut Oil

2 Organic Eggs

Natural Stevia, to taste

1⅓ cups Zucchini, peeled and grated

1 cup Almonds, chopped

Directions:

1. In a bowl, mix together the flour, baking powder, nutmeg, cinnamon, cloves and salt. In another bowl, add the oil, eggs and stevia, and beat until combined. Mix the egg mixture into the flour mixture. Fold in the zucchini and almonds.

2. Grease and flour a 2 pound coffee can. Transfer the mixture into the prepared can. Arrange the can in the slow cooker. Cover the can with 8 paper towels.

3. Set the slow cooker on high. Cover and cook for 3 to 4 hours.

Banana Strawberry Bread

The combination of bananas and strawberries *add the perfect touch of fruity flavor to this easily made bread. Serve with a topping of chopped nuts.*

Servings: 4
Prep Time: 15 minutes
Cooking Time: 3 hours

1¾ cups Almond Flour

¼ teaspoon gluten free Baking Soda

2 teaspoons non-aluminum, gluten free Baking Powder

½ teaspoon Flaked Sea Salt

⅓ cup melted Extra Virgin Coconut Oil

2 Organic Eggs

Natural Stevia, to taste

1 teaspoon Organic Vanilla Extract

3 Ripe Bananas, peeled and mashed

½ cup Fresh Strawberries, hulled and chopped

Directions:

1. In a bowl, mix together the baking powder, flour, salt and baking soda.. In a separate bowl add the oil, eggs, stevia, vanilla and bananas, and beat until combined. Mix the egg mixture with the flour mixture and gently fold in the strawberries.

2. Grease and flour a loaf pan. Transfer the mixture into the loaf pan and place the pan in a slow cooker. Cover the pan with 8 paper towels.

3. Set the slow cooker on high. Cover and cook for 2 to 3 hours.

HOLIDAY RECIPES

Creamy Lobster Veggie Soup

This rich and creamy lobster soup will be a great hit on any occasion. Serve with a garnishing of fresh lime slices.

Servings: 4
Prep Time: 15 minutes
Cooking Time: 8 hours, 45 minutes

---

1 cup Fresh Mushrooms, sliced

½ cup Fresh Tomatoes, chopped finely

1 Scallion (white part only), chopped

1 White Onion, chopped

1 teaspoon Dried Dill Weed

⅛ teaspoon Smoked Paprika

⅛ teaspoon Cayenne Pepper

Pinch of Ground Dry Mustard

Pinch of Ground Cinnamon

Pinch of Ground Nutmeg

Pinch of Ground Cloves

Pinch of Ground Allspice

Pinch of Ground Ginger

Flaked Sea Salt, to taste

Freshly Ground Black Pepper, to taste

4 cups Homemade Low-sodium Chicken Broth

2 Lobster Tails

½ cup unsweetened Coconut Cream

1 tablespoon Fresh Lime Juice

Directions:

1. In a slow cooker, mix together the vegetables, dill, spices, salt and broth. Cover the slow cooker and set to low, and cook for 6 to 8 hours.

2. With a hand blender, bled the soup slightly. Stir in the lobster tails. Cover and cook for 35 to 45 minutes.

3. Remove the lobster tails from the soup. Stir in the coconut cream and lime juice, and switch off the slow cooker.

4. Transfer the soup into a serving bowl. Top with lobster meat and serve.

Spiced Almond Chicken

This is a perfect dish for friends or family on special occasions.
Garnish with freshly chopped mint leaves.

Servings: 4
Prep Time: 15 minutes
Cooking Time: 6 hours, 6 minutes

---

1 tablespoon Extra Virgin Coconut Oil

2 small White Onions, sliced thinly

½ tablespoon Smoked Paprika

½ tablespoon Red Pepper Flakes that are crushed

½ teaspoon Ground Cinnamon

¼ teaspoon Ground Cloves

¼ teaspoon Ground Allspice

Pinch of Saffron

2 pounds (907g) Grass-Fed skinless, boneless Chicken Thighs

Flaked Sea Salt, to taste

Freshly Ground Black Pepper, to taste

1 cup Almonds, toasted and chopped

Directions:

1. In a skillet, heat the oil on a medium heat. Add the onion and sauté for 4 to 5 minutes. Add the spices and saffron, and sauté for 1 minute more. Transfer the mixture into a slow cooker.

2. Sprinkle the chicken with salt and black pepper, and add to the slow cooker. Mix the chicken thighs with the onion mixture.

3. Set the slow cooker on low. Cover and cook for about 6 hours.

4. Top the chicken with almonds and serve.

Cheesy Stuffed Chicken Breasts

Goat cheese and spinach along with herbs make a wonderful stuffing for the chicken in this recipe. Serve with fresh greens.

Servings: 4
Prep Time: 15 minutes
Cooking Time: 8 hours, 10 minutes

---

4 Grass-Fed skinless, boneless Chicken Breasts

Flaked Sea Salt, to taste

Freshly Ground Black Pepper, to taste

1 tablespoon Extra Virgin Coconut Oil

1 small White Onion, chopped

2 Green Chilies, sliced thinly

2 teaspoons Garlic, minced

½ cup Fresh Spinach, chopped

½ teaspoon Fresh Oregano, chopped

½ teaspoon Fresh Thyme, chopped

¼ cup Goat Cheese, crumbled

1 tablespoon Fresh Lime Juice

1½ cups Homemade Low-sodium Chicken Broth

Directions:

1. With a sharp knife, cut a deep slit into the center of each chicken breast to form a pocket. Sprinkle with salt and black before setting aside.

2. In a skillet, heat the oil on a medium heat. Add the onion and chilies, and sauté for 4 to 5 minutes. Add the garlic and spinach, and sauté for 3 to 4 minutes. Stir in herbs, salt and black pepper and cook for a further minute. Remove from heat.

3. Stuff each chicken breast with cheese equally. Now stuff the breasts with spinach mixture evenly. Arrange the breasts in a slow cooker. Drizzle with the lime juice. Pour the broth over the chicken breasts.

4. Set the slow cooker on low. Cover and cook for 6 to 8 hours.

Olives & Tomatoes Turkey

This amazingly delicious turkey dish will please every member of the family. Garnish with fresh lemon slices.

Servings: 4
Prep Time: 15 minutes
Cooking Time: 7 hours, 30 minutes

---

2 pounds (907g) Grass-Fed boneless Turkey Breasts

1 tablespoon Fresh Lemon juice

½ cup Black Olives, pitted and sliced

1 cup Onion, chopped

¼ cup Cherry Tomatoes, halved

1 teaspoon Garlic, minced

1 Fresh Oregano Sprig

1 Fresh Thyme sprig

Flaked Sea Salt, to taste

Freshly Ground Black Pepper, to taste

⅓ cup Homemade Low-sodium Chicken Broth, divided

1 tablespoon Arrowroot Starch

Directions:

1. In a slow cooker, add all ingredients except broth and arrowroot starch and mix. Pour half of broth over turkey mixture.

2. Set the slow cooker on low. Cover and cook for about 6 to 7 hours.

3. In a bowl, mix together remaining broth and arrowroot starch. Open the slow cooker. Stir in broth mixture.

4. Cover and cook for about 30 minutes more.

Tangy Salmon with Cilantro

This tasty and easy-to-make recipe of citrus ingredients
enhances the flavor of salmon greatly. Garnish with Lime slices.

Servings: 4
Prep Time: 15 minutes
Cooking Time: 1½ hour, 30 minutes

1½ pounds (680g) Salmon Fillets

½ cup Yellow Onion, chopped

1 teaspoon freshly grated Lime Rind

1 teaspoon freshly grated Lemon Rind

1 teaspoon freshly grated Orange Rind

¼ cup Fresh Cilantro, chopped

1 tablespoon Extra Virgin Olive Oil

Flaked Sea Salt, to taste

Freshly Ground Black Pepper, to taste

Directions:

1. Arrange the salmon fillets in a slow cooker. Top with all of the remaining ingredients.

2. Set the slow cooker on low. Cover and cook for about 1½ hours.

Spinach Bean Curry

This dish is easy to prepare and will be a great addition to your meal repertoire. Top with freshly chopped parsley leaves.

Servings: 4
Prep Time: 15 minutes
Cooking Time: 5 hours

1¾ cups Homemade Low-sodium Chicken Broth

1¾ cups unsweetened Coconut Milk

1 tablespoon Curry Powder

1 large Bunch Spinach, chopped

2 cups Fresh Green Beans, trimmed

½ teaspoon Ground Cumin

½ teaspoon Ground Cilantro

Flaked Sea Salt, to taste

Directions:

1. Mix together all of the ingredients in a slow cooker.

2. Set the slow cooker on low. Cover and cook for 4 to 5 hours.

Saucy Meatloaf Bliss

This recipe makes a fantastic and lavish meal for family gatherings on special occasions. Serve with fresh greens.

Servings: 4
Prep Time: 20 minutes
Cooking Time: 6 hours

For Meatloaf:

1½ pounds (680g) Grass-Fed Lean Ground Turkey

1 large Organic Egg, beaten

1 Celery Stalk, chopped

2 Scallions, chopped

½ Yellow Onion, chopped

1½ tablespoons Dijon Mustard

1 teaspoon Smoked Paprika

½ teaspoon Cayenne Pepper

2 teaspoons Dried Thyme, crushed

Flaked Sea Salt, to taste

Freshly Ground Black Pepper, to taste

For Sauce:

¼ cup Homemade Tomato Paste

2 tablespoons Dijon Mustard

1 teaspoon Smoked Paprika

1 teaspoon Fresh Lemon Juice

Flaked Sea Salt, to taste

Directions:

1. Mix together all of the meatloaf ingredients in a large bowl. Form a meatloaf from the mixture. Place the meatloaf in a slow cooker. Gently press to flatten the loaf.

2. In another bowl mix together all of the sauce ingredients. Pour the sauce over the meatloaf.

3. Set the slow cooker on low. Cover and cook for 4 to 6 hours.

Apple Almond Crisp

This is a perfect recipe in your dessert collection for special occasions. This dish is one that you may want to make time and again. Top with shredded coconut.

Servings: 4
Prep Time: 20 minutes
Cooking Time: 6 hours

---

4 Apples, peeled, cored and chopped

3 tablespoons Ground Cinnamon

2 tablespoons Almond Butter, softened

¼ cup Almond Flour

¼ cup Almonds, slivered

2 tablespoons Coconut, shredded and unsweetened

1 teaspoon Organic Vanilla Extract

Directions:

1. Arrange the chopped apples in a slow cooker. Sprinkle with 1 tablespoon of the cinnamon.

2. In a bowl, mix together the remaining ingredients. Pour

the almond mixture over the apples.

3. Set the slow cooker on low. Cover and cook for 2 to 3 hours.

14 FOODS LIST GUIDE

Here is a helpful guide of typical brain healthy and gluten-free foods for your shopping list.

1. **Healthy Wild Fish** such as: blue crab, sardines, shrimp, flounder, anchovies, sole, wild salmon and herring
2. **Non-starchy Vegetables** such as: cabbage, turnip, bok choy, broccoli, lettuce, mushroom, squash, cauliflower, cucumber, tomatoes, bell peppers, celery, onions, zucchini and green leafy vegetables such as: kale, spinach, mixed greens.
3. **Healthy Nuts** such as: almonds, walnuts, pecans
4. **Healthy Seeds** such as: chia seeds, flaxseeds, pumpkin seeds, sunflower seeds, sesame seeds
5. **Healthy Fats** such as: extra-virgin olive oil and coconut oil, grass-fed butter, ghee, avocado, shredded coconut
6. **Healthy Proteins** such as: grass-fed beef, organic pork, free-range chicken and turkey, free-range eggs
7. **Healthy Sugars** such as: low sugar fruits including limes, pumpkin, lemons, natural stevia, berries, cantaloupe
8. **Healthy Vinegars**: balsamic vinegar, raw coconut vinegar, apple cider vinegar
9. **Healthy Starches**: arrowroot powder, coconut flour, almond flour, flax flour
10. **Healthy Cheeses**: most cheeses can be eaten; however, cheeses that contain gluten such as blue cheeses should be avoided.

11. **Healthy Condiments**: Avoid processed condiments such as ketchup or catsup and stick to homemade, gluten-free and low-sugar condiments instead.
12. **Healthy Beverages** such as: filtered water, organic unsweetened coconut water, organic unsweetened almond milk, organic unsweetened coconut milk
13. **Natural and Organic Herbs, Seasonings and Spices**
14. **Salt**: Flaked sea salt, coarse sea salt or regular sea salt

Bear in mind that this is not a conclusive list and simply represents food items on a typical gluten-free shopping list.

LET'S COOK IT SLOW!

Without a doubt, the health benefits of living gluten-free are undeniable. Moreover, by merging gluten-free cooking with the slow cooker you'll be able to prepare almost every imaginable meal from appetizers to desserts. With the simple recipes and procedures in this cookbook, you will know exactly how to successfully create healthy, flavorful and convenient slow cooked meals—all gluten-free.

My journey into the gluten-free world started with my diagnosis of poor memory recall at only twenty-one years old. I had failed to alleviate my symptoms with prescription drugs, and finally decided to eliminate grains, gluten, refined sugars and heavy carbs from my diet. Consequently, I strongly believe that if living gluten-free has improved my health, then it is quite likely that it will improve yours too. As I tell everyone, I will never go back eating wheat and grains. Oh no! The rewards of living gluten-free are far more precious than any food temptation. So join with me and let's cook it slow—for even better health.

Thanks again for choosing my book. If you find this gluten-free slow cooker cookbook to be helpful, I would appreciate if you would let other readers know about it. I hereby wish you all the best in your quest to improve your brain's health. Live a healthy life—eat gluten-free!

Yours in health,
Sheryl Jensen

19453154R00126

Made in the USA
Middletown, DE
20 April 2015